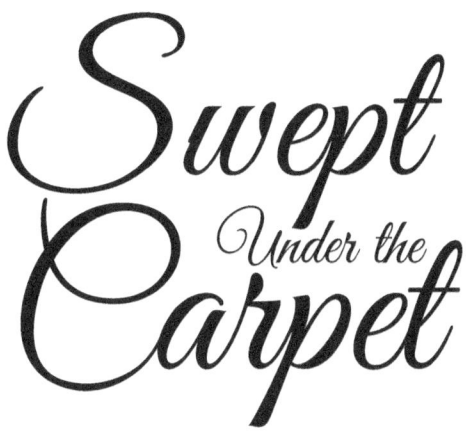

Swept Under the Carpet

A Personal Journey of Distress, Connection, and Healing Pre- and Post-Hysterectomy

Carmel Schleger

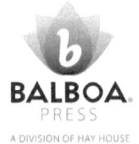

BALBOA
PRESS

A DIVISION OF HAY HOUSE

Balboa Press books may be ordered through booksellers or by contacting:

Balboa Press
A Division of Hay House
1663 Liberty Drive
Bloomington, IN 47403
www.balboapress.com.au
1 (877) 407-4847

Print information available on the last page.

ISBN: 978-1-5043-0432-0 (sc)
ISBN: 978-1-5043-0433-7 (e)

Balboa Press rev. date: 05/30/2017

Contents

Acknowledgements

$\mathcal{I}$ wish to take this opportunity to say thank you to those who helped me as I faced my personal challenges and also as I worked on this book:

- My family members particularly my dear mother Rose, through her wisdom and experience of such an ordeal gave me sound advice; my partner Noel; sons Tristan and Brendan, Noel's sister Sharon and dear friends who supported me through my entire hysterectomy experience—the process and emotional journey. Just them being there and listening to me was so very helpful.

- Dr Patricia Sherwood (PhD, Graduate Diploma in Special Education, B.A. (UWA), Graduate Diploma in Arts (counselling), BSW, Diploma in Holistic Counselling, Advanced Diploma in Holistic Counselling, Diploma in Buddhist Psychotherapy and Counselling, Diploma in Training and Assessment Systems, Graduate Certificate in Artistic Therapies; AHHCA, ACA, AASW,

Accredited Mental Health Social Worker) College Director and Principal of Sophia College and her educators taught me skills that became tools I drew on as I healed and returned my body, mind, and spirit to a state of well-being.

- Receiving healing energy and unconditional love from my two "wascles," my pets, Jimmy and Raffie, was a blessing and very much an important part of my healing.

Sadly, as I finished writing this book, my darling miniature poodle, Jimmy, passed away on 24 March 2016. He was the most angelic gentle pet I have ever had, and will always remain in my heart. Thank you, Jimmy, for being there for me. I will miss you.

I wish to acknowledge the traditional Elders and Owners both past and present of this land where I live, work and play

Introduction

Wow! Thank you for picking up this book! For you to do this, you must have gone through the process of a hysterectomy or are facing one. Or you may know someone who has had one or is going to have one. Because of this, you have witnessed, perhaps, an emotional change in either yourself or the person you know.

The idea for this book and the information I provide are drawn from my own personal experience. I am not an expert in this field. I am not a doctor or a psychologist; however, I chose to outline my whole experience: how my emotions were exposed and raw and what steps I took to reclaim my life, my identity, and particularly, *my body*. Not every woman reacts the same way emotionally upon hearing the news that she requires a full hysterectomy. In fact, for some it is complete relief, and they feel very grateful.

My specialist was quite considerate when I first shared with him my thoughts, concerns, and emotional state, even though he at first was quite taken aback that a woman of my age was so upset. (I was not sure what he meant by that!) Keep in mind that, whether he was or was not aware of the holistic impact on my being, I still felt obliged to share with him the huge emotional blow the news had on me.

I deeply encourage you to seek appropriate specialists in the field in your area and ask as many questions as you need to. Verbalize the feelings and emotions you may be experiencing to the professionals involved so that they are aware of the impact this procedure is having on you. Basically, ask for help *when* you need it.

Validate your emotions because they are real for you. Women are not the same, and we each experience this major procedure differently. Recovery is a personal, individual experience, and healing time varies.

In this book, I share my experience and how I chose to take control of the situation and self-nurture myself back to being a motivated woman, enjoying life again.

I also share the activities and therapies I used to assist me in regaining strength, self-worth, and vitality. Because I am trained in holistic counselling, art therapy, emotional literacy, and life coaching, I had the skills to self-coach myself through this ordeal. However, when I needed support, I did seek it. I am not an artist; I have no training or qualifications in how to paint or draw. The drawings I have shared in this book are expressions of my emotional feelings. As an alternate tool, I used the activities of art therapy to release the pain in a more creative, sensitive way, rather than having to verbalize it. Using this method, I was able to recognize the emotion and connect with it, and then slowly and gently work through it to begin my release.

I have also included some information on simple art expression exercises that may help you as well. However, if you are under the guidance of a mental health practitioner,

I encourage you to consult with him or her first before you attempt any of these activities.

Woman! The feminine have the capacity to create, generate, and nurture another human being. It is a gift to be honoured. However, due to health circumstances, a well-performed hysterectomy can cure a disease, save lives, or make life more comfortable. Whatever the reason for your drastic invasive procedure, I hope this book provides helpful guidance particularly with the emotional impact of the surgery as you prepare for it and as you recover. I trust you will gain some comfort that you are not alone, your emotions are normal, and there is support. There are also many things you can do to validate and honour your body, in particular your uterus, ovaries, hormones, bladder, and any part of your body that is affected by surgery. God bless them and you.

Carmel

The Reasons for a Hysterectomy

I begin my story with these questions: What is a hysterectomy? And why is there an increase in the number of women who have to go through the procedure?

Technically, a hysterectomy is the surgical removal of the uterus, or womb. Sometimes the fallopian tubes and ovaries are also removed.

There are different reasons this surgery is advised. The perceived medical reason could vary: a prolapse of the uterus or bladder (which appears to be a symptom of vaginal child birth), fibroid tumours, endometriosis, cancer of uterus and ovaries. These are just a few of the possible reasons, and each of these conditions can be a shock in itself.

Because all women are different, as are their medical conditions, there is simply no single remedy that will physically or emotionally assist every woman pre- or post-operation. Variables also include age, fitness whether she has given birth or wants to and I was told that a hysterectomy would be the solution for my medical issue. The bottom line is that I made the choice to have the surgery. There was history of a female family member who'd had cervical cancer and this, was for me, the most governing factor for my decision. So this, as well as other issues, were the deciding factors in my choice to have the procedure. However the sound medical evidence still did not ease the emotional response I went through. It was as if I had made the decision from the logical, analytical left side of my brain, but the creative, intuitive right side of my brain had not caught up. Another way of putting it is to say that, basically, the left and right sides of my brain were not in sync and I was torn in the decision making.

Perhaps if you are having a hysterectomy because of more sinister medical reasons, your emotional response may be filled with more hope and relief. If that is the case, believe me, I am right there with you in spirit. I am praying that it is successful and will contribute to your further good health and well-being.

My own story is honestly relayed here in this book from my personal perspective. I hope my story helps all women who may have similar experiences in their own personal and emotional journeys.

Chapter 2

My Story

This has been a very private and personal event in my life. However, travelling down this path overwhelmed my senses and awareness, and "I"—as I know "myself"—was altered. I experienced an overpowering emotion regarding my identity as a woman and what it meant to be a woman, To have been blessed with the capability, if I chose, to create another life, then to nurture it and incubate the many stages of pregnancy. I was transported to a place where I had never been before and found myself on an emotional and physical roller coaster for which I was not prepared.

My choice earlier in life had been to be a mother, and I had been blessed to give birth to two sons. On reflection, I thought of the women who choose to have children, and due to some unforeseen reason, they miscarry or are unable to conceive. As a woman, my heart goes out to you. I expect that, in these situations, women make choices to connect emotionally to the expected journey. They most assuredly start to build dreams—dreams that biologically may never come to fruition.

After being told that, because of my prognosis, a full hysterectomy was the best option for me, I surfed the Internet for sites and for links to books that could give me information to help me understand what I was feeling, what was going through my mind. I was more interested in this sort of information than I was about information on the procedure itself.

In all my research up to the time of writing this book, I have not found a reference about validating the feelings and emotions that can accompany this major invasive operation—the removal of the female reproductive organs—the "female bits." There may be a book or some related comprehensive information on the emotional "fallout" since I have written my story, but up until now, there have been none, or rather I have not found it easy to locate one.

Thankfully, as I am a trained holistic counsellor, life coach, and art therapist, I was able to recognize the emotional trauma that began on the day I left my specialist's rooms after having been informed that a full hysterectomy and further corrective surgery for other organs of my body would improve my well-being. Well, here I was, my gyno had just given me the news that, despite the corrective surgery that I'd had four years previously to repair, with mesh, a prolapsed uterus and bladder, I now needed a hysterectomy. He provided me with dates and a preparation schedule and I suddenly found myself on an emotional and physical roller coaster for which I was not prepared.

I know I was in touch in varying degrees with so many emotions. There were many different intensities to my awareness and I felt that it was necessary to highlight the impact on my whole being. I felt again I needed to validate for each and everyone one of us the effects of the procedure on each individual, which manifest in so many different ways.

Something's afoot—disbelief and shock

In June 2014, just before I had my regular women's health check-up with my general practitioner (GP), I began to feel a sensation that there was something not right. It was very uncomfortable and it felt too familiar. Similar to my previous prolapse of the uterus and bladder which was repaired four years previously. This as a result of having given birth to two babies vaginally. It is a pretty full-on statement to begin with, I know, but this is the story of the journey that I have been on and how it silently all but consumed me. This was not something I was prepared for; indeed, no woman is prepared for it. Does anyone speak openly to anyone about this sort of thing? This is so personal and private. Being "abnormal" or "different" in such a personal part of the body is something that is not usually a part of everyday conversation. Even while I am writing this, I am cringing at my descriptions and what I am writing about, but what pushes me along to share my journey is that too many women around the world go through this. We must understand that any perceived dysfunction of her reproductive system, externally or internally, can emotionally affect any woman. Women deserve validation and they deserve to be listened to. All the emotional support needed should be available to them.

I moved my appointment forward, as I thought I'd best get the symptoms looked at. Recognizing the sensation and discomfort, which I had previously experienced a few years before, I began to experience that sinking feeling of dread rise up through my chest and radiate up into my head, giving me a sense of being unbalanced and wanting to topple over.

Surely not, I thought. I grappled with the thought that the corrective surgery I had undergone four years before may have not been as successful as expected. *Please, please let it be just some other type of women's discomfort that can be fixed by the application of an ointment of some sort.*

No such luck! My GP, who is a petite young woman and very gentle, after the routine pap and internal examination, looked at me with understanding big brown eyes. Without her even verbalizing the fact, I just knew that my organs had prolapsed again!

As she confirmed the condition, my GP sat me down and advised me that I would need to see a specialist who could give me information about my options. As she scanned my face as I sat there, she picked up on my disappointment. She advised me that she could write a referral to a specialist who had a surgery not far from hers, just a suburb away. Listening to her and still having that sinking feeling, I felt my shoulders cave in as a sense of dense weight landed on on them. I felt quite defeated. That sinking feeling returned and now churned in my stomach area. I nodded my head slowly. "That would be good," I said, as I did not feel at all connected to the specialist who had conducted the previous surgery. I needed someone who had more empathy and consideration and would appreciate my needs. With the referral in hand, I felt somewhat shaky in my legs. Leaning on her desk for support, I stood up and bid her goodbye with a smile pasted on my face. I made my way to reception to pay for the consultation.

Having finalized the consultation bill, to maintain some balance, I cautiously turned slowly away from the reception desk and focused on moving towards the door. Gripping the door handle to steady myself, I manoeuvred through the door and out into the sunshine. On reaching my vehicle, I took a deep breath and gave myself a pep talk: *It can't be that bad! What I will do I will just go along to the specialist and see if he can do a little nip and tuck, and then everything will be apples!*

Hearing the words play out in my head, I felt a little bit better. I wasn't going to "buy into this". Taking a deep breath, I slid the key into the ignition, backed out of the car park, eased my way out around the traffic islands in the medical centre, and headed home.

Four months further on

With life being busy and my own business keeping me on my toes, I postponed the specialist visit—probably too long, now that I look at it retrospectively. Playing mind games with myself, I thought, *If I keep busy and pour all my time and effort into work, the problem will one day just automatically and miraculously be sucked up, and everything will be back to normal.* But then, *Yeah right! Who am I trying to kid? Carmel, are you deluded?*

In fact, the longer I left it, the worse it got. Finally, it got to the stage where I could not postpone seeing the specialist any longer. Life presently was stressful with family issues and busy with client needs. I also had a lot on my plate managing my elderly parents' personal needs. You see, that is what I do and what I am good at—looking after other people's needs and putting them first. Mmmm ... But the message I was finally getting was loud and clear: *Hey, girl, get yourself to the specialist now!*

October had arrived, and also the day of my appointment with the specialist. As I sat in the waiting room, I flicked through a mothering magazine, which didn't really resonate with me. Finally, the door opposite my chair opened, and there stood in front of me is a very tall man. He said hello to me and gestured me towards him. I quickly looked at his hands and made a silent gasp. I walked through the doorway, and my specialist gestured to a seat opposite him. I smiled and handed over to him my previous records and a copy of the referral from my general practitioner. My new specialist was very courteous and told me a little about himself and what he specialized in. He had already received a copy of my referral. Looking at me with a likeable smile, he asked me to tell him, in my own words, the symptoms I had recently experienced. He also asked me to tell him a little about my previous operation. While I spoke, he jotted down some notes, all the while nodding his head and occasionally looking up at me to establish eye contact.

Having listened attentively to me, he advised me that, to get a better understanding of the situation, he would need to do an internal exam. *Oh no!* I thought. I knew he had to, but the exam itself would confirm that the whole thing was really happening. I was about to get final confirmation about my condition. *Where's the door? I want to get out of here!*

He stood up and moved forward to open another door for me. He gestured me to enter. *Oh dear, this isn't the exit I wanted! This is the examination room, and, struth, look at that "rig" I have to sit on!*

I'll spare you the details of the examination, as I probably have already lost some readers who may have chosen to throw the book into the bin! But carry on. I will share my story for the sake of all the beautiful women on this planet who have to go through this medical procedure for the sake of their physical health and well-being.

After the examination, my specialist discreetly left the consultation room to allow me to tidy up. It was soon time to meet him back in his office. *Well, here we go*, I thought. *What is the prognosis, please?*

My doctor made some notes, intently looked down at his records, and slowly looked up at me. He began to talk, and I sensed that I was beginning to feel rather faint. His voice began to sound a tad distorted. *Oh no! Am I going to faint?*

I took in a deep breath, straightened my back, and with a jolt I was back and present in the room. It was just as I had thought—the previous procedure had been unsuccessful. This specialist just confirmed that for me. During my previous surgery, surgical mesh had been placed and hooked strategically in my body to keep my vital organs in place. The mesh was supposed to prevent these organs from prolapsing towards the vagina, putting pressure in the area. (Oooo, just writing this I feel so exposed! *Carry on, Carmel! This needs to be voiced for sake of all women! Deep breath, front and centre!*)

The mesh must be replaced, the specialist informed me, but for it to work even more effectively, a full hysterectomy would be beneficial. Hearing this, I leaned forward in my chair with my jaw and head held forward. *What?* I thought. *Does he want to remove* EVERYTHING?

I made contact with his eyes and searched them for some clarity as if I had received the information incorrectly. With a pen in his hand, he moved a large brochure across his desk so I could see it. Referring to the illustrations in the brochure, he proceeded to indicate what needed to be done. I was "gob smacked" by the number of pictures with very long descriptions and some very long words under them. He began to circle certain passages to show me what he suggested was necessary. *Oh no! I am beginning to feel very faint again! This meant removing everything!*

Sitting in a state of disbelief, I could feel tears brimming in my eyes and my bottom lip began to involuntarily quiver. *Carmel, remain dignified please.* I listened to my internal dialogue. *Who am I trying to kid? There is no dignity remaining for me or any other woman or maiden who needs to have these procedures. The doctors are going to remove the essence—what makes me a potentially fertile, creative, nurturing, reproductive female, a hormone-charged, awesome, empowered machine!*

At this stage I verbalized to my specialist that I was feeling overwhelmed and sad. As he folded his hands in front of him, he leaned a little forward over his very neat clean pristine professional oak desk and in a low voice blended with warmth in a matter-of-fact manner said "For any woman of your age with these previous issues this is the best option".

Suddenly, when I heard those words *your age*, I was jolted again out of the strange space I had retreated to! *What did he just say? Come again?*

I looked down and stared at my hands as they gripped my handbag. I was sitting forward on the edge of the chair suspended in time and space. I asked, "What has age got to do with it"? With sensitivity he advised me—and this is my recollection rather than his exact words—that once a woman has gone through menopause, her ovaries are no longer required or useful. Removing them would prevent possible ovarian cancer and that would benefit my well-being.

Whoa! I took a deep breath and remained calm and collected. *Hmmm. Okay. I see where he is coming from. So this is also a preventative measure and could possibly save me from having ovarian cancer.* I could appreciate what he was saying and I understood it on an intellectual level but my "being" on the whole, just could not get around all of it. I valued his honesty and perspective. At that stage it just didn't fit where I was right then and there. Still reassuring me, he continued to mention further preparation times and dates. On that note, I found myself levering myself out of the seat and we began to bid each other a good day.

Somehow I managed to navigate myself out of his consultation room to his receptionist to complete transactions, organize dates for further tests, and book into the hospital. I may add that I managed to do this in a jovial manner and even crack a joke. (I should have been a comedian!) Finally, with all those formalities completed, I courteously said goodbye and gazed around for the front door. *Ahhh! My composure is slipping. I need to get out of here!*

The front door at the entrance of the specialist's rooms finally closed behind me, and I was out in the summer sun and heat. Without fail, I began to feel quite detached from my body, as if I had been catapulted into space. It was surreal! I dragged my feet, and my whole body felt so very heavy. Finally, I reached my vehicle. Standing unsteadily there in the heat, I fumbled around in my handbag for the ignition key, finally unlocked my car door, plonked myself down in the driver's seat, and unconsciously placed my hands over my tummy. Tears began to well up in my eyes.

Here I was, a woman in my late fifties—closer to sixty than fifty years old. (Oh, yuck! When did this happen?) The emotion that washed over me was overwhelming. I realized I was in shock and in disbelief that at this stage for me to have a more quality of life, this procedure was the way to go. Sitting quite still in my vehicle and not really aware of the still-warm air in the cabin, I stared blankly over the car park. Then I heard a voice coming from within me. *What is going on here? Is this for real? Does this procedure really need to be done?*

I was totally shaken. I knew from my training that my "spirit" had disconnected from my body and had taken off above me to hover in a safe place. In fact, just typing this and relaying the experience to you now has once again catapulted my spirit out of my body. From my training I know that the terminology for this phenomenon is *excarnated*. With self-encouragement and long deep breaths, I feel a little bit better. I can now reconnect my whole self and will continue to share my experience.

Time was moving on, and I finally become present and aware of the smothering heat encompassing me in my reliable four-cylinder motor vehicle. I automatically wound down the windows to allow fresh air to flow. Still in that place of neither here nor there, I continued breathing and tapping my arms and hands to bring myself back into my body and be present, which had to happen before I could reverse out of the car park and merge into the traffic. *Where do I go?* I couldn't even remember if I had another appointment or if I should go home.

I decided to stay put for a while, have a swig of water, and splash some water over my face. That helped a little. At this stage, I decided to call my partner, Noel, as I knew he would be waiting with bated breath to hear the outcome of the appointment and to find out how I was feeling. As soon as I heard his level, empathic, calming voice, I began to cry. Between sobs, out of nowhere, a wave of memories and emotion came over me. I was taken to a place where I hadn't been before in this capacity. This place was where I felt isolated and a tsunami of emotion overwhelmed me. It was the place where I began to mourn. Within that split second, my whole being was awash with the processing of sadness, grief, and loss. Reality hit me, and I realized that I had an emotional attachment to the parts of my body that made me uniquely a woman. This attachment was increased because of the importance I had placed on the role these organs allowed me to carry out in life. I had felt so honoured to be able to conceive, carry, and nurture two children.

My partner really listened and I was able to compose myself a little. He suggested that I go directly home and rest. After our goodbyes and love you, we both hung up. It appeared to me that I placed my mobile on the passenger's seat beside me in slow motion. Even now, upon reflection, I can still see myself doing this. There is really no other way I can describe it except that it was like watching myself from a distance. *Whoa! Breathe, Carmel, breathe!*

Coming to the realization that I could not sit all day in the car park, I took Noel's advice. Eventually gathering enough composure to drive, I reversed out of the car park and merged into the flow of traffic. I was willing myself to be calm and present and to concentrate on driving. Somehow I managed enough composure to drive through annoying, bustling traffic. I continued to drive to the outskirts of suburbia and eventually through the cutting in the mountain, up and over, and back to my sanctuary of fresh air, peace, and quiet, back to the village just on the outskirts of the metropolitan area of Brisbane.

Eventually I make it home and slowly turned into the driveway of our little plot of paradise. I scanned our little property and felt a pang of gratitude. I eased up the driveway, as it is unsealed, and with no recent rain, a speedy approach would churn up the dirt and gravel, leaving me in a cloud of dust when I open the car door to get out. I slowly pulled up in front of the house and saw through the glass pane at the front door a tiny little fluffy face with his nose pressed up against the glass. I gave him a little smile, even though he would not see it. But my smile of acknowledgement for him seemed reassuring to me. You see, my devoted elderly miniature poodle, Jimmy, was sixteen years old, deaf, and blind. In addition, he had a canine cognitive dysfunction that caused him to become trapped in areas of the house. He had trouble finding doorways, didn't respond to his name or commands, and had the onset of dementia among other problems. I believe he felt the vibration of the car coming up the driveway, so habit brought him to the door. Whatever the reason, it was nice to see his little face at the door to greet me.

Feeling really flat at this stage after receiving the news of my pending procedure and concentrating on my long drive home, I finally dragged myself inside, acknowledged and gave a cuddle to my Jimmy, and greeted my oversized, affectionate ginger cat, Raffie. I found my way to my bedroom where I flopped onto my bed. Resting my head on the not-so-comfortable pillow, I sank into the folds of my mattress and, on cue, the floodgates of emotion opened and tears flowed. I was back in that state of awe I'd been in a few hours previously, caused by test results and the matter-of-fact conversation with my specialist about what was going to happen to me and the parts of my body that made me female.

Allowing the tears to flow, I lay there in silence and stared up at the ceiling. I'm not sure how long I did this, but finally noticing the moistness on my cheeks and the fact that my nose felt it needed to be clear, I broke my stare leaned over to the bedside table and reached for the box of tissues. After mopping up tears and clearing my nasal passages, I remained resting on my bed. I found I could not fathom that this procedure had to be done. Thoughts of *if*, and *but*, and *why me?* were circling through my mind, and I continued to lie there with a blank look on my face. I suddenly felt a sense of presence in the room; I became distracted. I gazed over the side of the bed my two "fur kids" standing side-by-side, looking up at me with such concern and love in their eyes. Once the ginger cat, Raffie, caught my eye, she somehow sent a signal to aged, blind Jimmy, and they both instinctively jumped onto my bed. They lay by my side and rested their heads on my tummy. Lying there with these sweet, innocent, unconditionally loving pets by my side and sensing and feeling their empathy and care, I was so grateful that the tears began to flow again.

I then resolved that I would simply allow myself to feel these emotions and not trivialize this experience. I would honour myself in doing this. Having made this decision, I felt a little lighter, and emotionally exhausted, I nodded off to sleep.

Chapter 3

Whirlwind of Emotions

I was relieved and pleased that my pre-op appointments and consultations were happening later in the year. During this time, my business appointments were winding down in my position as a consulting counsellor and life coach for a number of job service providers. It certainly would not have been a pleasant situation trying to handle a large caseload when I was personally in a fragile position.

As I mentioned earlier, I finally came to the realization that for me to heal, this major operation would, indeed, have to happen. I then gave myself permission to feel all of the emotions that came to me. At this stage I was not really certain what other emotions were going to surface. However, being a holistic counsellor for some years had helped me to understand that there would be layer upon layer of varying emotions and I would probably feel a number of emotions all at once. And I would probably feel a number of emotions all at once. There is no hard and fast rule to this; each one of us processes his or her emotions at a different rate. It is when the emotions linger for many, many months and you find you are paralysed by this emotional burden that it is recommended that you seek ongoing professional emotional support either as an individual or in a group support environment.

Over the following weeks, my emotions were all over the place. I kept thinking about the day of the procedure, my time in hospital after the operation, and then six to eight more weeks after that during which I would be unable to do anything but rest at home. There was no particular order to the range of emotions that showered over my total being. The intensity and length of time I experienced each emotion varied greatly. However, I feel I need to share with you the complete emotional turmoil I experienced. If you or someone you know must go through this, or have gone through this, be reassured that by feeling, honouring and healing the whole encounter, *you will come through the experience, and you will be able to function.*

As I prepared for the forthcoming surgery, my body responded in a way that held up the surgery date. I had to go for further tests and treatment for an unrelated condition. Be mindful that this is also a possibility for anyone facing surgery of any kind. Your body might react this way as well. Whether it was out of sympathy or a method to stall the procedure, I became extremely backed up and bloated. It was as if my body was trying to control and hold onto everything and anything. I was in extreme discomfort, and further tests had to be explored before my scheduled hysterectomy. In the long run, these tests were done and completed. Reflecting on this occasion, I feel that these were physical symptoms of stress. *No more false starts.* The date was confirmed: Tuesday, 30 December 2014, in the afternoon.

Sadness, grief, and feelings of loss

These emotions were constant from the beginning, as soon as I received confirmation that the operation was going ahead. They lasted for several more months after the surgery during my recovery. I felt so sad. There was no vitality or cheeriness in me, and I sensed that I was just dragging myself around like a wet blanket. I withdrew from the world around me and did not venture out much from my home. I felt I needed to do that to allow myself to feel this emotion and see it through. Those who lived with me honoured me in giving me the space to do so. At times, out of the blue, I would start crying. I would profusely apologize, but with the support of my partner and complete understanding from my dear friends, I felt I was being suspended in a safe environment where I could succumb to the relief of the tears. With each cleansing tear I shed, I kept reminding myself that I was one step further along the road of healing.

In an article posted to the *Psychology Today* website on November 26, 2011, Marc Bekoff, PhD, wrote, "Grief in itself is something of a mystery, for there doesn't seem to be any obvious adaptive value to it in an evolutionary sense. It does not appear to increase an individual's reproductive success. Whatever its value is, grief is the price of commitment, that wellspring of both happiness and sorrow."

Sadness is, to me in this moment of time, an element that is attached to grief and loss. Upon receiving the news that a full hysterectomy would be the solution for my discomfort, and that it would improve my well-being, I still was overwhelmed by grief that the surgery had to occur.

One day I was at home sitting in the family room staring out the double glass door overlooking the backyard. I began weeping for the inevitable loss of my womb. This was the place where, after being conceived, each baby had been protected and embraced. It was the babies' incubator, keeping them nourished and warm until it was time for them to be born. It was a part of me, and each child had been born of me. My womb was their first home. I mourned the loss of the only connection I had left to the one I had miscarried. In my head at that time, I could only connect my physical body parts—especially my womb—to the memory of the beginning of my babies and how unconsciously significant this was to me. For me the connection of mind and body and, in this instant, the connection of my mind to my reproductive organs was so personal that I could not separate them; they were totally as one.

I grappled with these thoughts and cognitively tried to rationalize them. How could I rationalize an unconscious feeling that was so intense? Again, my hands automatically and gently placed themselves on my tummy in a protective manner. My tears again were flowing, and it felt as if they were being transported up and through my whole body. It was totally surreal. It felt as if my life as I knew it was at the beginning of a transition, and I would be different from that moment in time.

Drawing on my training, I was aware that the imprint of the cellular memory had been stirred, and in order to begin healing I should embrace my skills and express the experience in art.

The household was quiet, and I was home alone. Being totally present with the moment, I took myself off to a quiet place, located crayons and paper, and sitting quietly, with my palms gently placed on my abdomen, I breathed in and out gently. With intention, I allowed my mind and body to travel into that area of emotions and to sense the quality of what and how I was feeling.

Whilst sitting there, I allowed the crayon and colour to command what to draw. I didn't let my mind contribute to or control the process. I proceeded to engross myself in the flow and expression of the feelings of loss and sadness through art.

Suspended in this emotion, I allowed colour and shapes to unfold onto the paper in an artwork of expression. I felt my divine feminine grieving not for just myself, but for all women who have gone through or will have to go through this incredibly invasive surgery—the removal of her "creative energy portal". When I came to the realization that this procedure—this hysterectomy—happens to hundreds of thousands of other women in every country over the globe, I felt that I needed to express this in its totality. I then felt the urge to acknowledge each and every female human as well all female animals who have this procedure. I affirmed that each female is a magnificent, courageous, strong, and majestic being. Being in this space as complete expression poured out over the paper and the energy swooned through me, I felt more space open up in me. It was so expansive and connected to the female energy that my heart felt it was going to explode with gratitude and empathy.

I sat back in my chair and scanned over my piece. *Wow!* There was so much expression of emotion for universal female creative energy and for myself. It was my creative expression, and it was out of my body. I felt that my energy level was quite spent. The exercise had been so emotive, and the energy that was triggered in my body was electric. I felt tingling pulsing sensations through my limbs. *Wow, what a buzz, and it was all self-generated!*

After sitting glued to the chair for so long, I felt I needed to get up and move and assist the energy to pulse through my body without any blockages. Moving around, breathing deeply, and gesturing with my arms and body in flowing graceful movements I began to feel more grounded as the experience threw me out of my body just a bit! I then felt compelled to continue to do these moving exercises to express and validate the feminine energy of my own being and every female on this planet, reaffirming that we are incredible beings.

Reconnecting with my original drawing of grief and loss, I considered the qualities of the feminine energy. The terms that came to mind were: *caring, nurturing, loving, nourishing, inclusive, intuitive, receptive, creative, of unlimited capacity, accepting of self, contributing, demonstrative, mother, daughter, sister, aunty, grandmother,* and *elder* to name a few.

With this inspiration, I opened up to the quality of these words and was drawn to express my reactions in colour, swirls, and shapes. I created an abstract of the healing I had just experienced.

When I completed the piece, I leaned back in my chair, arms slumped and resting in my lap. Relaxed and spent, I gently began breathing in the colour and energy of the resource. I lazily scanned the creation—my art of expression—I had just completed, and without effort I felt light and clearer in my head.

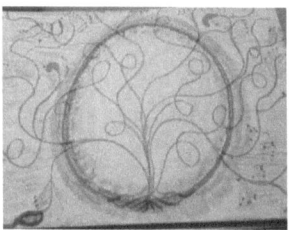

Anger

Anger can appear to be so distant from emotions that appear to be more delicate like sadness, grief, and loss. But anger is a very real emotion and can make itself known when you least expect it. A few weeks had passed since I had started digesting the reality of my impending operation. With the medical procedure constantly in the back of my mind, I was aimlessly pottering around at home, folding some clothes, and laying them out on my bed, when I became aware of an energy form that was getting more intense in my solar plexus. With this sensation, my breathing seemed to intensify, and I was aware of the muscles in my face and jaw constricting.

I sat down on the edge of the bed, looked down at my feet and thought, *Okay, Carmel, what is going on here?* I slowly looked up and saw my reflection in the full-length mirror opposite me and was confronted with what I saw. I came to the realization that I was annoyed and angry. Feeling this sensation intensify, I levered myself off the side of the bed. Standing up, I placed my hands on my solar plexus and breathed in. I sensed that I wanted to spew out the thoughts that were building up in my body, particularly in my midriff area.

I closed my eyes and asked myself, *What am I angry about?* At that time, clearly the answers came to me. I was angry at myself and felt that precious parts of my body had let me down. I also felt that *I* had let that part of my own body down. With a jolt, I opened my eyes and questioned, *Whoa, where did that come from?*

As I continued to breathe into the area where I could sense blocked energy in my solar plexus, I decided I had to release the pressure, so using knowledge from my training, I symbolically gathered the energy from around the area, and gestured that I was scooping the blocked anger energy up and throwing it out of my system. With the gesture, I grunted a sound "Grrrr ..." to help me disperse the energy. This eased the tension some; however, I came to realize that I would need to explore this further, as I had made a commitment to myself that I would not be a victim and that I would be a stronger, more empowered woman in all areas of my being—body, mind, and spirit.

It was time for me to take action. I did not want to feel this way. It was difficult enough to accept that this medical procedure was going ahead, and that alone was a mammoth invasion of my whole being. I had to keep moving and be as prepared as much as I could and work through the whirlpool of emotions that were threatening to drown me. I retreated to my bedroom where I had set up an artist's easel and paints in the corner near the full-length, free-standing mirror. I closed the door to keep the fur kids out of the room, as I did not want anybody—not even my pets—to bear witness to my activities and absorb negative energy that might result from the process I was about to undertake. I sensed I would be dispersing a lot of negative energy, and the expression on my face would probably indicate just how much.

Facing the easel with the colour pallet and brushes ready, I centred on that feeling of anger that was trapped inside my body. I was automatically attracted to colours of deep red and dark orange. I created violent coloured strokes and allowed my angry energy to be flung and etched onto the canvas. I felt myself immersed into the activity and channelled the anger from my abdominal area up through my arms and out on to the canvas. After I spent an intense, focused period of time releasing the anger from my body onto the canvas, I took a breath and stepped back. There, in front of me, was my anger, spurting out in outrageous colours from strong and purposeful strokes from my brush. No longer was it stuck like a solid block of energy in my body. No longer did I have the sense that I had let myself down or that my precious body parts had let me down. No more did I have a sense of interruption and inconvenience in my life and career. And no more did I have a sense of high expectation. It was out! I had expressed it!

Sitting down on the side of the bed, I gazed at the canvas and instantly felt a sense of relief. The energy block wedged between my stomach and solar plexus had finally been eliminated. I could feel I was breathing more evenly than earlier.

I re-evaluated my own good qualities and gave myself a hug whilst I stood gently rocking. I expressed appreciation for my courage to confront this emotion. I removed the art piece out of my room and placed it in my home office, face down on the desk. It was not something I wanted to view. It had served its purpose, and a few days later I thanked it and released it with appreciation, ceremoniously burning it. I created the version you see here by sensing into the memory of the experience and recreating the artwork.

Symbolically and personally, I let go and dispersed this intense energy out into the ether to be cleansed and purified by some divine positive power. The anger that raised its ugly head before the procedure has not returned.

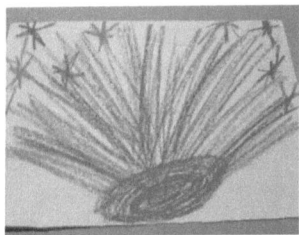

Betrayal and judgement

During the emotional, turbulent time leading up to the day of surgery, I discovered that in this toxic soup of depressing emotion, I had thoughts of betrayal of self. Betrayal is a core issue in the human experience. It can destroy relationships in intimate unions, in the workplace where there is betrayal between colleagues, and too frequently in society where there is betrayal of family members through abuse. In essence, I have learned through my training that it is an act of disrespect. It is belittling, and energetically it cuts deep into the whole person. For some, if it is not addressed and healed, it can lead to a dark state of the mind, involving hatred and revenge.

In my case, though, I recognized I had the feeling that part of my body had betrayed the rest of me—my mind and spirit. And also that my mind and spirit had betrayed my body. In bewilderment I sat down and questioned, *Where in tarnation did this come from?* This thought threw me for a sixer, so I decided to do something tactile. Hanging out the washing was the go!

This task may sound simple; however, with two determined animals wanting to go out and play in the flea-infested yard at this time of year when there has not been much rain and it is hot and humid, I had to have eyes in the back of my head to make sure they did not escape. Tricky, but for the moment it was a great distraction from my perceived personal betrayal.

Having managed successfully to hang out the washing without a pet escaping the house, I went back inside, poured myself a refreshing cool drink, and decided to write down some notes on this emotional dilemma I had created in my head. This little exercise of jotting my thoughts onto paper always removes the problem of thinking and also literally eases the pressure out of my head so I can work through an issue. I wrote down the words that came into my psyche about betrayal:

- *Betrayal of self?*
- *What does that mean?*
- *Where did this come from?*

Betrayal of self! I got it! It came to me like a flash as my inner critic revealed herself! Here "she" was working overtime and capitalizing on my state of emotional vulnerability. To address this emotion of the inner critic, I would conduct a holistic counselling session with "her." I would do a judgement sequence. However, here I would be facing the sucker on my own. *I can do this!*

Once I identified what was really going on, I was able to separate myself from it. As an observer, I decided to be brave and explore this further. I sat quietly and asked, *Where did this come from?* I cleared my mind as much as I could to see if any picture or thought revealed itself. What came to me were not a strong emotion as some of the others had been. Rather it was an awareness that I was being extremely hard on myself and had in general quite high expectations of myself. There were no old patterns that came to mind of instances of being judged. I was quite amazed to "hear" the voice of my inner critic trying to put "her" ten cents' worth in, telling me I was too weak to stop this situation. It did not make sense. I was aware of my inner critic's work, and was not fazed by what I had discovered. With a sigh of relief, I sat back and thought, *Yeah, I have slain two negative thoughts with one exercise—self judgement and weakness. Delete!*

Pondering on my own personal challenge of betrayal and my own inner critic I began to think of other women, particularly younger women who for some medical reason were in this predicament and who wanted to have children, but would not be able to. Putting myself in their place I felt such empathy. A perceived betrayal of her own body by a woman in such a situation could possibly be an emotion that would surface with intensity and would impact her emotionally, distorting her perception of what choices she had in starting a family, her relationship with her partner, and her perception of being a complete, whole woman. If this is your situation, I encourage you to seek professional counselling to work through this limiting and disempowering emotional state. This can help you to gain clarity and identify your options.

Stress

Was I experiencing stress? Ah … yeah—just a tad! We are all familiar in some capacity with how stress can impact our lives, and when you are waiting for a pending invasive procedure, there is a possibility that you will display signs that you are experiencing other stresses.

Personally, I recall that my appetite changed. Even though I knew that I should prepare my body by eating wholesome foods, I found myself reaching out for and stuffing myself with comfort food. I was aware that I was choosing this food, but somewhere in the back of my mind, I, for a time, did not want to change. I was making a mindful choice at the time, and I took responsibility for my decision, cutting myself some slack as there was a lot going on.

Insomnia

Insomnia was also an unwelcome visitor. Suddenly, in the middle of the night a number of times, my eyes would shoot open. For a moment I would be stunned, and then the thought of my impending operation would seep into my consciousness. If I could not go back to sleep, rather than tossing and turning, I would drag myself out of bed, walk into the bathroom, and from the tap cup my hand and have a drink of water. I would have a bit of a stretch and take few deep breaths. If insomnia lingered, I would read and it would soon pass. I would flop back into bed to catch a bit more sleep until daybreak.

As well as this, another component of physical stress I was experiencing was constipation. Additionally, my blood pressure was raised. These circumstances did prompt me to be more mindful of what food I was eating. I decided to drink more water and keep hydrated. As I practised more relaxation and mindful breathing techniques as well as taking some light exercise, my blood pressure decreased. These activities were connected to my "self-talk."

Mentally, I noticed I was forgetful, and my senses were dull. These were unwanted by-products of my circumstances. Deep breathing, walking around the house, stretching, and when it was not too hot, going outside and pottering in my vegetable patch—these were, at the time, the only methods I could pull together to help my mind adjust and carry on. Unfortunately I had an injured, painful right knee which kept me from going for walks that would have been more beneficial. Fresh air, a change of focus, and walking would have definitely helped. Occasionally I experienced crying spells and spurts of anxiety, but I just threw them into my great big emotional melting pot and collectively "managed" them with all the other feelings that were swirling around.

I was aware that I was choosing to withdraw from relationships. My partner and I live just outside Brisbane in Queensland, Australia, on a little patch of land in the country. We were definitely not in the heart of the city. This made it even easier for me to withdraw from family, friends, community, and general interaction—just participating in the human race. Quite often I would not go past the front gate for days on end. My partner and I were both aware that I was doing this. He observed this and raised it in conversation with me, but he figured I was the trained counsellor and decided not to say anymore; rather, he sat quietly on the sidelines and verbally prodded me when he felt it necessary.

In retrospect, I know that this withdrawal and isolation, if not addressed, could possibly foster another unwanted visitor—loneliness. If not monitored, withdrawal can lead to something more concerning; however, for me it was this loneliness that stirred up a dormant emotion called frustration. It is not in my nature to lack motivation or to not contribute in some capacity to society. Now that I think back, I realize that frustration was particularly noticeable a few weeks after I came out of hospital. I was bored with lying around, resting, doing crosswords, watching television, and basically being totally inactive. Recognizing my frustration was like a kick up the backside. I began planning and thinking and organizing activities in which I could contribute. I looked forward to eventually going back to work. I looked back on the past weeks of my emotional and physical journey and recognized the vulnerability that I had been drowning in, and I came to a decision: I had spent quite some time processing these thoughts and feelings, and I had taken note of the change in my processing. I became aware that I was near the opening of an emotional "dark tunnel." With this realization I began to feel lighter and more accepting of the whole journey.

A very wise person sent me a message that touched my soul and has been the wings to lift me up and to move along: "There has been a lot of sadness in your life. It is time to stop looking back and start moving forward." Reflecting on this was the push I needed to keep going. (You know who you are … thank you.)

We can linger in the soup of negative emotions and get stuck. If soup simmering on a stove is not stirred and watched, it thickens and can eventually get stuck on the bottom of the saucepan—burnt and not suitable to eat. We have a choice—stay in the soup, get burnt, and be no good to anyone, or observe, acknowledge our situation and our emotions, work at healing, accept what has occurred, and move forward with what we have.

Stepping up and addressing these emotions does not mean that you will totally conquer all of them; it simply means that you will acknowledge and validate your journey. Personally, I found that sadness would pop up every now and then, particularly when I had returned home and was resting. Lying on the bed or couch on my own, I had the time to reflect on this incredible disruptive emotional and physical journey, and no matter how much healing I do, there will probably be traces of sadness as I move on. It will be like any grief over the loss of a loved one, even the unconditional love and companionship of a much-loved pet. It may never go away; with time it will just become a little bit easier to live with.

Chapter 4

Taking Ownership—
Ceremony and Gratitude

In the previous chapter I gave you a snapshot of the emotions that I went through. There was no particular order to the experiences; I purely wanted to give voice to the fact that I had actually experienced all of that emotional reaction. My own journey opened my eyes to acknowledge that other women may have already had or will have the same sort of experiences. When I was in this situation, I began to turn the wheels that moved me forward as I began taking responsibility for my healing by being productive and grateful for everything in my life.

As I travelled through this emotional journey of acknowledging, healing, and eventually accepting that I needed and was going to have a hysterectomy, I felt I wanted to do something private and special, just between me and the memory of what I thought of as the essence of my physical womanhood. I decided to conduct a ceremony of giving thanks and letting go.

This is a personal thing, and for some is not necessary. It is a personal choice, and whatever you choose to do is okay. There is no right or wrong, good or bad in the way a person chooses to heal and move on in this or any other situation. For me, though I had been honoured to support other women through similar ceremonies. I too, wanted to honour and thank my "woman's bits". To do this I decided I needed to stand in front of the "altar of gratitude" and say goodbye.

When there was quiet time in the household, I retreated to my private room and began to organize the tools I required to perform this ceremony. Pensively, I began to look around the room, looking for objects that I thought would work well for this exercise of healing. Gathering the special objects together, I placed them to the side of the little coffee table, which I was going to improvise as my altar of honour. Taking a breath and with intention, I began the task of laying out a velvet cloth over the top of the table, smoothing it out and making the sides sit evenly around. I then, one by one, placed the various objects that depicted meaning to me on the cloth. I fiddled around with placement of each one until I felt it was in the correct and final position. Next I gathered some tea light candles and placed them on the cloth, arranging them until I thought they were all in the right place. Standing back, I scanned the altar and made several more adjustments until it all felt right. Finally, having the feeling that everything was in the right place, I turned out the lights, gathered up the lighter and proceed to light the candles. As I lit each candle, the room slowly filled with soft light, and my altar of gratitude and healing took on a meaning and entity of its own. Stepping back from the altar, I took a deep breath and just allowed myself to be completely centred in the moment. There was present, a small sense of angst. Coming to the decision to express my emotions and feelings, and to give myself permission to feel, grieve, and say goodbye is still a very confronting act. However, I had the urge that I needed to do this. It was like making a commitment to myself and giving myself permission to move forward. Next, in the centre of the altar, I laid my final drawing and placed around it other meaningful pieces.

Just recalling the process, I can sense the energy of what a very special and sacred moment that was for me. With dim lighting and soft relaxing music playing in the background, I had set the mood of the environment for this special occasion. Within the four walls of the room, there was a sense of sacredness. Centering myself, I took a few gentle deep breaths and proceeded to give thanks as I released my physical attachment to my "woman's bits".

Spontaneously, I recited: "For all these years, I have been a part of you, and you have been part of me. There have been times with unbearable discomfort and pain, and also the amazing times of being pregnant and witnessing my body stretch and accommodate the growing child. I am grateful ..."

As my final words were very personal, and each woman who is reading this will have her own personal thoughts, I have not included mine; however, I am sure that my words were similar or in keeping words of many other women.

After sitting with this energy for a while, energetically I said my goodbyes. Time passed. I am not sure how long I sat there, but eventually I drew a deep breath, knelt in front of the altar, leaned forward, and one by one blew out the candles, watching as each flame went out and the plume of smoke wafted up towards the ceiling. Slowly I got myself up to my feet and gently stretched, gesturing in front of the altar with my hands in prayer position. I bowed my head and slowly stepped back from the ceremonial space. With positive energy, I removed myself from the room, figuratively closing the door and moving forward.

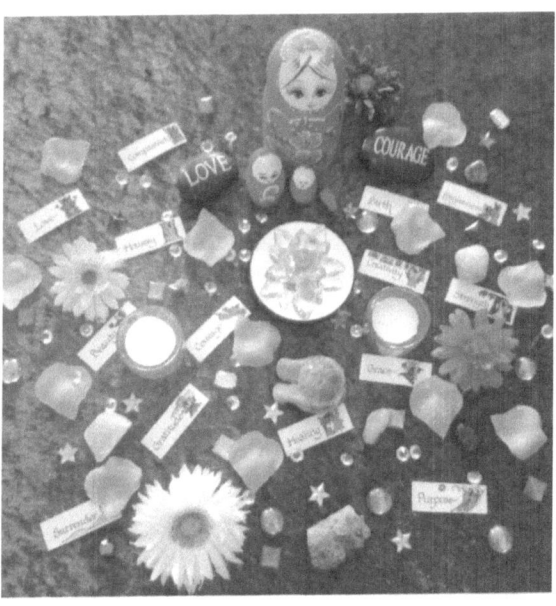

I felt I had experienced a death, which in a way it had been. It was the acknowledging that there would be an end to our relationship as we had known it and that after the operation and removal of "her," there would be an energetic and physical shift in the area of my abdomen. My life as I knew it would be different, and at that stage I was going through the motions of preparation. Further along we will revisit these emotions and sensations.

Chapter 5

Pro-Active Preparation

Practical tasks prior to hospital admission

*E*ven though I had spent quite a bit of time emotionally preparing myself for the pending hysterectomy, there were more practical things I needed to address. It was time to gather together the general things I would need in the hospital, such as toiletries, suitable bed clothing, and maybe a book and some crossword puzzles. The thing is, you probably will not use the entertaining elements, but it is handy to have them just in case.

It's a good idea to organize a support group to be there for you when you are discharged from hospital and return home. These people can assist you with household duties as well as support you getting in and out of bed if required. Just knowing that there is someone there for you is comforting, and it is most important to be receiving their gift of help to you. Generally, we women have a block on receiving from others. I say, receive it! I was blessed with two special people—my partner, Noel, and also his sister, Sharon, who was living with us at the time. She assisted me in every way. She took over all the household duties, cooked meals, and drove me to and from appointments. I truly accepted her gift with so much appreciation. The help they provided together allowed me the space and time to heal. To you both again—I thank you!

My adult sons, Tristan and Brendan, even though they were not living at home, were wonderful, loving, and caring in the support they offered. On hearing the news of my operation, they were quite taken aback, and they questioned why, as they knew about the major operation I'd had four years previously. They were truly concerned, and I could see in their eyes they felt quite helpless. They and their partners were incredibly supportive just with their random loving texts, visits to the hospital, and also visits regularly when I was recovering at home. For me, this unconditional love and support from family members and friends was the juice that gave me strength and the belief that all was going to be fine. I believe such support contributes to mental and physical healing and recovery.

With all medical operations, there is, without a doubt, a frightening element—the possibility of complications. Knowing that I was going in for major surgery, my awareness of my mortality came forward. This thought alone stirs fear and concern. I chose to face this feeling head on. When my partner and I were alone, I spoke with him. Later I spoke with my sons. I told them that *if* anything did happen, I had made an updated will. The thought of having this conversation can be daunting; however, having done it, I felt incredibly lighter, as if a heavy weight had been lifted off my shoulders. By doing this, I had faced my physical mortality. The payoff was the lessening of the energetic charge of another negative emotion from my mind. This allowed more space for healing energy and being positive. It was also comforting that I had faced the inevitable conversation head on. I felt that the conversation had taken my relationships with my family members to an even more special level of intimacy.

For the convenience of your loved ones, make a list of contact numbers of all family members and friends who wish to be updated on your well-being. Put it in an easy-to-find location, like the fridge at home, so that whoever is doing the notifying will see the list and remember to make the calls or send text messages. Doing this lessens the worry and stress of those around you, as they are, in their own way, probably anxious as well. You really need them present and centered when you return home, "sore and sorry," as the saying goes.

Personal well-being preparation

Leading up to the day of admission, I found it helpful to find time in my day to be still. Lying on my bed with my hands on my tummy I would breathe in and out, watching my tummy area rise and fall. As I did this, I would visualize a colour that I considered nurturing, caring, loving, and healing. I would imagine the coloured breath circulating through the area, bathing and soothing it.

By making the time to do this, I felt I was contributing to the preparation of my body, mind, and spirit, acknowledging that there would be physical changes after the procedure, and generally connecting and talking to my female organs, telling them that I appreciated them and would not forget them. Personally, I felt it was beneficial for me to experience as little stress as possible leading up to the day. This daily ritual became a very important part of my routine. It helped me to regulate my breath, be present in the moment, and let go any form of possible anxiousness.

As I prepared my personal toiletries, I included a bottle of lavender essence so that I could have a drop on a tissue to breathe in. It is a soothing aromatherapy oil, and sniffing it occasionally is like a refreshing breath for me. Another homeopathic tincture I used leading up to the big day was the Body Love System Organic Emergency Essence Mist, a product of Australian Bushflower Essences. I had this in the form of a mouth spray, and every few hours or when I thought of it, I sprayed some into my mouth. It has a calming effect and assists in alleviating the negative emotions of fear and distress. Keep in mind, I had investigated many modalities that would offer pre-operation well-being, and this was my own choice as I prepared for the operation. I have been familiar with Australian Bushflower Essences for many years and resonate to the natural healing properties. There is another similar essence Bach Flower Remedies Rescue Remedy Natural Stress Relief. I am not here to endorse any particular product; I just want to share with you in this book some of the ways I personally and emotionally prepared to cope.

There apparently is evidence, based on quantum physics, that the universe is made up of energy. I am a person who lives a life of energy awareness. I have run workshops on this topic. For example, have you ever been somewhere within a group of people and your inner knowing (your inner sense) informed you that you did not want to stand next to a particular person? You gently step away from that person. Without thinking, the message and response were inbuilt mechanisms of your senses—your whole self— picking up that person's energy and saying, "Hey, I don't want to be next to that person! That person is creepy."

As well as that natural, inner reflex, there is a variety of energy disciplines such as acupuncture, esoteric chakra puncture, and dry needling, to name but a few, that assist with the unblocking of energy, or chi, as the Chinese call it. So where am I going with this? Well, I chose to energetically prepare my body. I undertook several sessions in esoteric chakra puncture to unblock the energy of my body and to keep it flowing. For me, it was an amazing experience, and I did feel the benefit. I also had several sessions with a friend of mine who is an acupuncturist.

Massage was another part of my holistic preparation for my hysterectomy. I wanted my body to know that I was there for "her", that we were one, and that I was doing everything possible I could to stimulate happy feelings and to release any tension in my body. This is the great benefit of relaxation techniques. Before going to sleep, I would gently massage my abdomen with body lotion, continuing that connection to my sacred area. For me generally, I felt I was contributing to my holistic preparation and being proactive.

Keeping hydrated, having a daily bowel movement, and doing light exercise were beneficial as well. Talking to my body was a regular occurrence. I kept telling 'her' how much I appreciated and loved 'her'. I assured 'her' that we would come through this procedure eventually physically, emotionally and spiritually buoyant.

Here we go … night before prep!

Before I knew it, days and weeks had passed, and the time had come. It was the night before the life-changing op! I now had to begin the process of evacuating my bowels in preparation for admission.

Oh dear … here we go! What a night! Up and down out of the bed to make a run to the toilet. I finally gave up at one stage and decided to just sit on the loo for a while to try and get some sleep. Sleep lasted for a whole thirty seconds, but I was appreciative of the miniscule precious thirty seconds I did have, believe it or not. Just having not to frantically run to the toilet without messing myself was a small blessing. Hours passed, and at about four in the morning, I discovered that the frantic desire to run had passed. I actually fell asleep gratefully when my head hit the pillow. But before I knew it, it was daylight! Even though I was hopelessly tired and I felt physically empty, I actually was wide awake with an unmistakable clarity.

The day had arrived, and now there was no turning back. This was the day my uterus and I would be separated—unceremoniously, I might add. As I lay in bed, I felt I had done as much as I could to prepare for this event, and in a way I felt numb but resolved. The operation was going to proceed. It was a weird sort of place to be, and, yes, I will say I still felt some trepidation. But the inevitable was going to happen. Getting out of bed, I swung my legs to the ground and sat for a moment, taking a breath to psych myself up. *This is it! No turning back. Once I am off this bed, I will robotically get ready and complete packing my bag. How strange and out of place I feel.*

Chapter 6

My Stay in the Hospital

Arrival and preparation

The three of us arrived at the hospital—my partner, his sister, and I. As we pulled into the car park at the entrance, the three of us were very quiet. When the car came to a stop, I slowly levered myself out of the four-wheel drive and allowed my legs to slide down until my feet landed firmly on the road. For a moment I stabilized myself whilst holding onto the car door and taking a deep breath. In the meantime, my partner turned off the ignition, got out of the vehicle, and came around to my side of the vehicle carrying my overnight bag of essentials. Gently he said to me, "Come on, dear."

Quietly the three of us walked together into the foyer of the hospital. Before I knew it, I was standing at the admissions desk filling out the necessary paper work and receiving directions to the "gyno" ward. It was so dreamlike going through the motions. I turned towards the other two, and we started on our way. After we entered the lift to descend to the ward, we just stood quietly facing the lift door, obviously each of us immersed in personal thoughts. When I stepped out of the lift, I saw in front of me the long corridor, which I knew I had to walk down. For a hospital, it was incredibly dim and gloomy. I had a flash in front of my mind's eye of the movie *The Green Mile* in which the convicted prisoner's character, John Coffey, takes his final walk. A shiver shot down my back, and I once again coached myself to be calm. Even so, with each step towards the ward I experienced an element of anxiety. To be honest, a hint of fear became lodged in my throat. Again, I gently took a deep breath and regained my composure. I looked over at Noel and thankfully sensed he was oblivious to the angst and mind games that were happening within my mind at this time. Taking a right turn, we encountered another corridor to walk. Thank goodness it was nowhere near as long as the first one. There, I felt weird and, in a way, quite alone. We finally reached the reception area of my ward, and I felt relieved when we were welcomed by a friendly nurse who led us down yet another corridor to my room.

For me, this nurse was a blessing. She was jovial and light hearted, which changed the energy of what was going on inside me and what I perceived my partner was feeling. His sister, with a gentle heart and quietness, stood in the background and was just "being there" for both of us.

After the nurse gave me some instructions, she left the room. I stowed away my personal belongings and sat on the bed. Before long the cheerful nurse was back again wielding a razor. In her upbeat manner, she gave me instructions. I was aghast that I was expected to struggle, twisting my body to reach *that* part of my body, and with a sharp implement in my hand, no less! What the …? How is a woman in her late fifties, carrying probably a few more kilos than desired (that's right—I am voluptuous) going to accomplish a circus contortionist's act with a razor without ending up like the little Aussie TV personality, Norman Gunston, who used to do a comedy routine with tissue bits stuck all over little cuts on his face? And adding to that, what about the itchiness of regrowth! Ugh! Well, this was quite a contrast from the comfort I had been feeling a few minutes before.

Reluctantly I entered the bathroom. Rolling my eyes back at the other two, I closed the door behind me. It was frustrating just doing this exercise, but it was even worse to be aware that my partner and his sister were just on the other side of the bathroom door listening to me grunting and heaving heavy breaths as I expended energy on the task, focusing on not having an accident. Enough blood was going to be shed in the next several hours during surgery!

Finally I completed the task, and may I add, no blood was shed and a smooth job was done, despite the fact that I felt like a "plucked chook." I dressed in the required ensemble: a rather breezy hospital gown, the back held together (sort of) with only two flimsy ties, and a lovely pair of regulation pressed paper panties! I was now just waiting to be wheeled into the theatre.

I had actually welcomed the distraction of having to prep myself. It took the edge off the trepidation that had been building up within me and around me. Looking at my devoted, caring partner, I sensed he felt quite helpless, in that there was nothing he could "fix" for me. He didn't know how much it meant to me that he was giving of his time, that his caring nature was soothing to me, and that he would be there waiting for me when I came out of surgery. Moments like these reinforce the connection and commitment we have for each other, and his caring nurturing qualities always come to the fore.

Journey to the theatre—whoa, here we go!

Within minutes, the time had arrived. A nurse bounced through the door, followed by a wardsman. "Carmel, it's time!"

Noel came over to my bed, leant over, and gently kissed me. His sister, Sharon, also hugged me. I barely recall him saying that everything would be all right and that he would be there waiting for me when I came out of surgery. I barely recall mentioning the list I had left with him, and asking him to call, in particular, my two beautiful sons, and anyone else on the list to keep them all in the loop; otherwise, he would probably be inundated with many calls.

No sooner had we said, "Catch you later," than my driver, the wardsman, unlocked the wheels on my bed and began pushing me out the door. I looked back and, before I knew it, we turned right, and my loved ones turned left, and then were out of sight. Mr. Wardsman had to make a few tight three-point turns to manoeuvre me and my bed around a row of newborns' cribs that were lined up in the narrow corridor outside my room. Being chauffeured past I had started counting the cribs. I thought, *It must be quiet in the delivery rooms. Then maybe they are expecting quite a few babies to be born in the next few days with all these cribs lined up and ready to go. How ironic,* I thought, *being pushed passed these clear Perspex baby cribs all made up with mattresses and fresh, crisp sheets.* I stopped counting them after eight. I changed my gaze to the direction I was being wheeled. In front of me at the end of the narrow corridor I glanced through the open doorway of a private room and witnessed a new mother gazing down and caressing her newborn. Her partner was sitting beside her on the bed looking lovingly down at the little human that they had created together. It was such a beautiful site. It stirred an emotion in me that was actually a sense of joy for them and was also a confirmation of the cycle of life. How miraculous is it that we women are created with a womb—a sacred space that was made to protect a new human form from conception through to birthing. Wow, my bosom swelled with a sense of achievement that I had been blessed to contribute to the cycle of life.

That chapter in my life had been finished many years before. Now I was at the end of the timeline that included conceiving a child, nurturing and protecting the unborn in my womb, giving birth, having monthly periods, and going through menopause. My female organs were no longer necessary; indeed, they had become a hindrance to my general health and well-being. I lay on my hospital bed on wheels. The wardsman told me that the theatre was some way from my ward, and he said, "Enjoy the ride." *Enjoy the ride?* I just smiled to acknowledge that had I heard him and then slipped into a dreamlike state. Whilst being pushed along the corridors and in and out of lifts, through my semi-glazed eyes I observed several people looking at me. Some people offered up a token smile. Some were busy looking at medical records. I could hear babies crying in the background and the sounds of banging food trays. It was so surreal. My life as a woman who chose to have children, to carry them in my body, to nurture, love and raise them, was ending, and that day would be the beginning of the next stage of my life. Goodbye and thank you, dear uterus and ovaries!

Still gliding through corridors on my bed on wheels, I felt as if time had slowed down. The inevitable was going to happen soon, and I would wake up feeling sore and knowing things had changed. *Unless I leap off the bed and make a run for it!* But, even though I had not been given any drugs yet, I was out of it! Realizing that the surgery was really happening, I willed myself to be calm. I began to call on my spiritual beliefs—to pray for protection and courage whilst I was under anaesthetic and during the procedure. I asked my Creator to keep my whole being safe, and I asked that my dad, who had passed, would look out for me. In my mind, I reaffirmed my respect for myself and my body so that no negative-energy imprint was left on me.

Destination: theatre—no backing out!

When we arrived at the theatre, the wardsman pushed my bed into the waiting room just outside the theatre. Straight away, a nurse in full theatre garb began to ask me questions. The usual—full name, date of birth, and what type of procedure was I having. Whoa! I advised her that, at this stage, I did not recall the correct medical terminology for the procedure. "But in layman's terms," I said, "a full hysterectomy and corrective surgery and new meshing to support a prolapsed bladder." That appeared to be a suitable answer. I had no sooner finished answering her and then two other nurses introduced themselves and asked the same questions. Even though there was a tad of anxiety rising in my chest, I thought, *Well at least we all know why I am here and exactly who I am! It's comforting that we are all on the same page—well ... same theatre at least.*

At this stage, my specialist appeared next to my bed. He gave me his big friendly smile and said hello. He said I would be okay and he would see me in the theatre. Oh ... okay! Well, at least I knew he was doing the procedure. Throughout the preparation and visits with him before that day, I had shared with him the emotional conditions I had been experiencing since receiving the news. He was open to listen; however, I did feel he was quite perplexed at times that a woman of my age would be so emotional and so attached to her uterus. I don't think he had encountered this before. I had been quick to tell him, with diplomacy, that no two women of any age—regardless if they are over fifty—will have the same response or reaction to the news that they need a total hysterectomy. That is because no two people on the planet are the same, let alone two women. I compared it to two blokes getting the news that they required prostate surgery. I do not think they would receive the news or view the consequences equally! Well, that is my perspective, and it is my story, and that is how I could not see the relevance.

I do give him credit. The thing is, he listened and noted and validated that I was experiencing these feelings and emotions, and he did thank me for sharing this information with him. In a way, I had perhaps contributed a little more information about women and their feelings and emotions. I let him know that I believe how important it is for us to allow ourselves to feel vulnerable.

The time had finally come: I was wheeled into theatre. The first thing I noticed was that the temperature was so cold and the room itself was so clinical. When you think about it, that is a good thing. The staff got me to shuffle my body over to a very narrow bed. I felt I could easily roll off anytime, and I hoped they were aware I am not a size ten! I made the move as gingerly as I could because I was very conscious that the back of my garment was held together with a thread of a tie and I was wearing paper panties! For heaven's sake, I knew that everything was going to be bared, but at least I wanted to keep a skerrick of modesty alive, at least whilst I was conscious.

In the background I could see a number of theatre staff unpacking the surgical implements. I could hear them clang onto the pristine metal trays. To my left the anaesthetist interrupted my examination of the room and introduced himself to me. Again I had to rattle off who I was, why I was there, and my date of birth. To save myself from being pricked a number of times as they searched for a good vein, I told him that the right arm was an easier one to try. While he was talking to me, I took one last look around. I was just saying another prayer to my Creator asking him to look after me when … zzzzzz.

Chapter 7

The Deed Is Done!

What time is it? Is it all over? Really, is it all over?

$\mathcal{O}$ut of the darkness in the back of my mind, I could hear from afar someone calling my name. "Carmel, wake up now." I sluggishly tuned into the voice, and with great effort and strained concentration, I willed myself to open my eyes and try to scan around the room. Straight away, I felt my eyes close shut. I thought, *Oh, how I wish I could just go back to sleep! Leave me alone!*

But there was a knowing in the back of my mind that I had to wake up, hence I gave a big effort to will my eyes open. This time I was able to get through the blurry vision and see that there appeared to be quite a few people in the room. I must have been a sight to be seen. Through a foggy veil I could see my sons' faces. They seemed aghast to see, yet again, their mum coming out of anaesthetic after a major operation. Seeing their astonished faces, I made an effort to try and speak some sense to reassure them. It obviously did not come out right, but that was probably a good thing, as it lightened up the room when they responded with a nervous laugh over whatever I had said or tried to say. Noel came over and kissed me. Then it was the boys' turn. Over to the side of the room, I saw my eldest son's girlfriend sitting down. I think it must have been quite comforting for her to be able to sit back out of the way, as only twelve months before, her mum had been through chemo for breast cancer. I hazily looked at the clock and saw it was nearly six in the evening. Gosh, I been under for more than four hours?

Well, I thought, *so far I can't feel anything.* I wanted to lift up the covers and check out my tummy, but thought better of that. I decided to leave that for another time when the family had left. Besides, my arms felt as heavy as lead, and I was still very groggy. I gestured to everyone and said in some gibberish language that I was okay. Noel translated and told everyone they could go home. I could feel that they were still worried and did not really want to leave me, but with a very wobbly hand, with tubes and monitors still attached, I gestured for them to leave and forced a smile on my face to reassure them. *Mum is good*, I tried to telegraph to them. *Go home!*

Rest and road to recovery

On cue, the night shift nurse came in, adjusted and checked tubes and monitors, and asked, "How is your pain?" *Pain? What pain? Am I suppose to be in pain? Nah … there is no pain!*

It was all good at this stage! She advised that she would visit again soon and show me how to use the self-dosage mechanism that would help me with pain management. *Self-manage pain medication? Whoa! This is going to be interesting.* How am I going to know when to administer it? Well, I worked that out pretty quickly, may I add. Pain sure did reveal itself convincingly.

My visitors, including my sons, left finally. I told them that there was no need to come across town to visit, as I would be home in a few days. Besides, the next day was New Year's Eve, and the traffic around the city would be horrendous. My younger son offered to spend the arrival of the New Year with me. *Awww, how thoughtful!* I declined that offer, as I did not want him sitting with his mum and Noel looking at four walls and wondering what his girlfriend and friends were doing. I think, just between you and me, that he was relieved that I said, "No, thank you."

After all visitors except for Noel had gone, I had a little bit of dinner, and after the nurse came in to do "obs" (vital signs!) and administer more medication, my body and I were really wanting to go to sleep. Noel saw that I was tiring, quietly kissed me goodnight, and left. Welcome sleep! My body felt sore and stiff. Before lights out, I carefully raised my blankets and my nightgown and tried to look at my belly. I felt tightness in a number of areas, but I was still too groggy to lift my head further off the pillow to have a really good look. I slumped back onto my bed and thought, *Well, it's done now, and presently I feel no actual pain. I am ready for sleep.*

I vaguely recall, during the night, a nurse coming in with a torch, asking me questions, checking and restocking the fluids in the drip bag hanging to the right of me, and administering additional medication. Apparently I answered correctly, and without hesitation I nodded off to sleep once again.

The morning after

Before daylight, I found myself waking up. I think it was a sense of tugging and tightness in my abdomen that initially stirred me. The sensation brought me back to reality. I took a deep breath and thought, *Wow, it is all over. My women's bits are no longer a part of me.* I felt a sense of awe and sadness, and I lay there quietly with that sensation. However, I felt as if those two emotions were carefully wrapped in a blanket of practicality. *Carmel,* I told myself, *the decision has been made. The deed has been done, and you, girl, have to centre on health and recovery.* It made sense …

Ouch! Where is that painkiller? On cue, the morning shift nurse was in, checking all the paraphernalia attached to me, asking pertinent questions, and administering painkillers. "Thank you, thank you!" I exclaimed.

Without further ado, this "morning nurse" advised, "After breakfast, we will get you up and out of bed so you can have a shower and get into some fresh clothes!"

I thought, *Oh, okay. That sounds like a plan!* I actually was keen to get up on my feet as I was not going to allow myself to buy into a self-pity party. There was no chance that I would have the pleasure to even consider it. Even with thoughts of this up-front, matter-of-fact response going through my head, I still could sense in the background a sadness that my beloved reproductive organs were no longer nestled in between my made-for-baby-bearing hips.

They were gone, no longer physically a part of me. Feeling my nose begin to tingle and tears beginning to bead in the corners of my eyes, I let the sensation wash over me, but this time I took another deep breath—a great thing to do in a time of crisis—and willed myself back to be present and to concentrate on my body, which really needed to be the centre of attention for the proper nurturing and healing of one who has gone through so much emotional and physical trauma.

Okay here we go … let's get off this bed! *Whoa! Pain! Ouch! Ouch! Bl*#dy h3ll! This hurts!*

Flopping—gently—back onto the bed, I recalled that, to get out of bed after surgery, the best practice is to roll on your side and push with your arms. Then you can centre yourself for a moment before levering yourself up. *Okay, here we go again. Let's try it.* Well, I did that slowly and carefully. Finally I was sitting on the side of the bed with my feet hanging over. I took a few breaths and proceeded to stand on the floor. *Ouch, ouch, oooouch! What the? Thought I was on painkillers? Why is the top left-hand side of my belly sooooo painful?*

I could not straighten up at all. Here I was standing hunched over and favouring my left side.

I eventually make it onto my two feet. I leaned forward and to the left a bit to ease the localized extreme discomfort. Eventually I did the "granny shuffle," barely lifting my feet off the floor. I felt extremely vulnerable, and I had no confidence at this stage in my balance and coordination. Very slowly I made my way to the bathroom door and shuffled in. Directly in front of me I saw in a large mirror the reflection of a very drained and tired-looking older woman. *Oh, that's right—it's me! Struth, I look terrible!*

I actually sometimes forget that I am much older than what I *think* I am, and today was an unfortunate confirmation that, yes, I am an older woman who has just gone through the mill! *Oh well, them's the breaks!*

At least I knew that, through the monitoring of the nurses, being fed, resting, and taking plenty of painkillers, each and every moment that passed brought me one step closer to recovery.

Now, down to business—strip off. Or I should say slowly and painstakingly remove my simple garment. I took a warm shower, washing my body, including my very wild and bouncy hair, which had looked very drab and well slicked down over my cheek. Finally I was able to lower over my sore, bent body my own fresh, clean, brand-new nightie! How nice to be rid of those garments that are left gaping at the back! Whoah! This took quite a bit of effort; however, I felt much better already. That warm shower of water cascading over my pitiful beaten-up body had been heaven!

Feeling in a much better frame of mind and a little energized, I opened the door to find my dearly beloved sitting quietly in the corner chair. He smiled as he watched me waddle across the room towards the bed.

Chapter 8

A Few Days After

Discomfort and moving forward

*S*everal days had passed. I'd been pricked and poked, given pain killers, and had my blood pressure being checked. My mood was picking up; however, the excruciating pain in my left side would not give up, regardless of pain numbing medication.

I would not allow this discomfort to deter my conviction to keep moving. Each day, every few hours, I would lever myself off the bed and move about my room. With each step I was feeling my balance come back, and I began to feel somewhat stronger and a little more confident. When I finished my effort to keep moving, I would return to bed, and automatically my thoughts would go back to the major procedure I had just gone through. Regardless of the progress I was making, and the fact that, on the outside,

I *looked* strong and resilient, I was still hovering, lost in the emotional space. Regardless the amount of emotional preparation I had done beforehand, I still experienced remnants of sadness, grief, and loss. I had to acknowledge that these were not emotions that were just going to go away! My emotional discomfort was still lingering; I just could not give it the full attention it required as I had to focus on my physical well-being so that I could be discharged out of hospital in reasonable physical form.

Whilst resting in between visitors and nurses doing observations, I regularly would place palms down over my tummy, gently rest them there, and allow the warmth of my palms to radiate into my abdominal area, just to reaffirm to me and my body that we were connected and that through nurturing and gentle steps we, as a team, would work towards wellness. This was a very important gesture for me to do. It helped me keep *connected* to the whole of me, as the whole of me was affected—not just my reproductive area. The procedure had impacted the whole of my being. Staying connected to my whole self opened the door for the whole of me to begin to recover and heal.

My specialist popped in daily to measure the success of the operation. He told me that, from his personal perspective, he was very happy with everything. He advised me that I could go home in the morning after only two days. This suggestion, however, I declined. Even though I was picking up, the gripping discomfort and pain in my left side had not diminished, and my gut feeling (excuse the pun!) encouraged me to stay longer. Also, seeing that I had been paying private insurance all those years, I figured that I had Hospital Cover, and I was going to take a couple days more, just to make sure all bits were working reasonably well. My specialist was supportive and said, "Stay as long as you want!" And I thought. *Thanks. I will!*

In all seriousness, I wanted the b!**dy pain in the top left-hand side of my tummy to dissipate before I packed up and left. I actually really wanted to be back at home and receive some unconditional "pet therapy"; however, I just had an inkling that I needed to stay a little longer.

It turned out that my gut feeling was spot on. Even though the side pain and pulling had not dissipated, I woke up the next day coughing up little blood clots. This, I may say, frightened me. I questioned myself, *What are small blood clots doing in my throat?*

As soon as a nurse came into the room, I showed her. Immediately, she advised that she would go and get the doctor on shift. Within minutes, the intern came and checked me out and reviewed my medical file to see if this was at all related to my operation. Deep in thought, he left the room; within an hour he returned with news for me. It was confirmed that there were issues with the tube that had been inserted down my throat by the anaesthetist. The tube had inadvertently scraped the inside of my airways. There was another unrelated concern that flared up from being in surgery, but that can be left for another story of my life.

The follow through by the intern and the attending nurse who reported this slight setback at the time was commendable. Their quick response and action was comforting and gave me some relief and confidence.

Even though I was improving physically, in tiny baby steps, when I was not distracted, a silent ripple of sadness would again wash over me in the form of gentle slow tears sliding down my cheeks and the block of energy that formed in my chest and throat.

Nurse Hope

Whilst being in this state of energetic disruption in hospital and needing to release the pressure valve of my feelings, intuitively I shared what I was holistically experiencing with a lovely young nurse who had an aura of empathy and compassion. Instinct encouraged me to verbalize my emotional journey through this hysterectomy. I shared with her my experience and told her that I considered it a blessing that I had been trained in counselling and art therapy and that I was able to address at intervals the feelings that would surface. I explained my awareness that there did not appear to be much recognition for the fact that women do experience overwhelming feelings of distress. For the sake of the story, I will refer to this nurse as Nurse Hope.

This lovely young nurse responded with complete understanding. She validated my feelings and told me that she had witnessed other women suffering not just the physical pain of the hysterectomy, but also the emotional pain of separation and disempowerment. She confirmed my thoughts that there was no readily available emotional support for such women of any age. As well as that, she was aware of lack of empathy in the medical field. Many professionals were not capable of understanding. In saying this, we as women, are not criticizing the perceived lack of empathy; rather, we are validating that there is a need for such empathy, and because it is not readily available, we understand that specific counselling would certainly assist in the healing of the physical and emotional trauma. A referral service could connect patients with such counsellors.

Our conversations were confirmation that my intuition to get the word out there was of utmost importance. I needed to help people understand that what women of all ages experience and feel is *real* and not to be pushed aside with a sweeping statement such as, "There will be depression for a while, but you will get over it." Is this supposed to be supportive? Well, it certainly is not empathetic! This statement is not a reflection on anyone in particular. It is what I have read generally in well-being articles on many health websites.

I believe there must be a holistic approach to health. All aspects of a woman's health—physical and emotional—should be taken into consideration with regard to a hysterectomy, whether it is a full or a partial procedure. As well as emotionally feeling grief, loss, and sadness, there is also the physical impact of hormonal changes, which also contribute to emotional wellbeing.

From my chats with Nurse Hope, I learnt that there was another woman, a little younger than I, who'd had the procedure a day after mine. We communicated through Nurse Hope, each enquiring how the other was coping. That alone was comforting for both of us; even though we never met, we looked out for each other.

Information I gained from my conversations with Nurse Hope, together with my own thoughts and personal journey, further convinced me that there was a need to bring attention to the fact that the emotional trauma to a woman having health challenges that inevitably led to a hysterectomy is real and needs to be validated and addressed with empathy and counselling to assist with healing.

Unfortunately I did not get to say thank you to Nurse Hope and to wish her a wonderful life. She really was a sweet young woman and had amazing energy about her. If you, Nurse Hope, find this book in your possession, thank you again.

Time to check out of this place

Well, another day or two passed, and still the strange pulling and the pain in my left side had not dissipated. The medical staff showed no real concern or explanation as to why this was happening. One nurse did say that it was possible the internal stitches in that incision might be extra tight and could be causing the discomfort. With that explanation in the back of my mind, I thought that I really had had enough of my hospital stay. I decided then and there to check out!

I woke up early, showered, and began gathering my personal belongings together, so that when my doctor came to visit, I would be ready and waiting to leave. Finally, all my "obs" had been checked and my specialist and nurse had signed off. No sooner had they left my room then with upbeat enthusiasm, I was on my "mobie" calling my knight in shining armour—my dear partner, Noel. "Come and get me. I'm coming home today!"

When the patient service attendant came in to collect my breakfast tray, I wished her a good morning and, in an upbeat fashion said, "Hi! I won't be here after brekkie, as I am going home today!" Now I am not sure if she heard me or she really didn't care, but there was no actual response to my happy exclamation. I was hoping for a *"That's nice dear. All the best"*. Rather than this I sensed her response would be more like, *"Yeah, heard that before. Bet you are going to be here for morning tea at least!"*

You know what? She would have been right! At around ten o'clock, she came to the door still with a deadpan look on her face and asked, "Morning tea?" *Well*, I figured, *if I am here, why not? Another cup of tea, a slice of cake won't do too much damage to my widening girth!* Wrong! I learnt the hard way. A little advice here, girls—monitor what you are consuming daily. As the weeks passed, I was eating and not exercising, and I personally felt that the extra weight did aggravate the healing process of my internal scars, as even today I still get a twinge and a twang every now and then.

Noel had advised me that he would be there after ten. Sure enough, after my morning tea, he arrived. "I see you're already packed and ready to go," he said.

"Sure am," I said. But I hadn't seen a nurse since earlier that morning, and here I was thinking, *Hey, I wanna go home. When do I get the all clear and a wheelchair so that I can get to the car in style and without any pain?*

No sooner had that thought crossed my mind than another nurse came in with a bag of medications and a list of instructions for taking them. When she was finished explaining everything to me, she advised that I could leave. I said, "Is that it?" She said yes and told me that, if I had any concerns or worries after I was discharged and at home, I should just call my specialist.

Oh, okay! I thought. *Bugger! No wheelchair! Do they have any idea how far it is from this ward to the entrance of this hospital?*

64

I was hoping for a pain-free ride to the foyer, as there were a number of flights of stairs to contend with. (Would you believe it? The lift from my ward to the next level was out of order!) I became light-headed from the exercise of gripping onto the rail, stepping cautiously from one step to the next, all the while pressing firmly the left side of my abdomen where the pain from the internal stitches was still growling at me. Considering that I had not been mobile at length for the last five days, and had been predominantly flat on my back, here I was now waddling down the corridor where baby cribs were lined up against the wall in a neat row. Managing to stay reasonably upright was a right old struggle. How ironic!

Noel grabbed my overnight bag and flowers with one hand and my arm with the other hand. In his quiet empathic tone he coaxed me: "Come on, dear." I looked up at him as I slouched over, caressing my very tender left side, and I actually think I dropped my bottom lip like a sulking little child! We shuffled down the hallway, past all the baby cribs. I noted there were fewer there, maybe meaning that several more babies had arrived into this world. *How nice!*

We eventually reached the nurses' quarters, which doubled as reception for the ward. I looked for a familiar face so I could say goodbye and thank you, but I saw only one familiar face. She was the nurse who had not been very friendly at all, and she was looking down at paperwork in front of her. In fact, I sensed that she might have been completely over it all. Well, when you think of it, she looked around my age, and had probably been doing this gig for over thirty years. I guess for some it would be a challenge to keep up the facade of engaging with each and every patient who wants to say hi. But then you, never ever know! She too may have had worries that lay heavily on her mind and totally absorbed her attention. Well, fair enough. The other two nurses there had their heads together engrossed in what I perceived as a patient's file. One of them gazed over at me with no particular acknowledgement at all and then continued talking to her colleague. *Oh well! I am really just another number—I mean another woman who has had a traumatic, invasive surgery! (Sigh). You know-when it comes down to it, I am so thankful for nurse's caring and monitoring my progress. Where would we be without them?*

We finally reached the bottom of the stairs, and I needed to pull up to catch my breath. Patient Noel stood there, and with encouragement, placed pressure on my elbow to keep moving. In my head I hear myself say, *Suck it up, Carmel! Let's go!*

Next came the soft-shoe shuffle down a very long corridor passing many patient rooms, nurses' desks, bustling staff members, and visitors to wards. Even this effort of moving closer to the main entrance of the hospital was a most surreal sensation. I felt as if I was in a movie scene in which the lens scans the faces of people from the perspective of the actor walking forward.

Second stage accomplished. We made it to the other lift, which would take us up to the foyer of the hospital where I would see daylight, not through glass windows or in the comfort of air conditioning. There I would get the full impact of the heat of the sun all over me, and the humidity would swirl around my body. Bliss to feel ... well, for a minute at least.

Having thought of everything, my partner propped me up against a post near the drop-off bay and trotted off to his car. When he brought the car to my waiting place and jumped out, I realized that, as usual, he had thought of everything. He had brought a portable step for me to use, which lessened the stretch I needed to make to lever myself from the ground up into the large four-by-four truck. As I sat there after all that extended effort and with limited oxygen in my lungs as well as feeling the heat from the sun, all I could think was, *Quick, hon! Crank up the beast and turn the air-con on!*

Chapter 9

Home Sweet Home

The journey home

*A*s we left the grounds of the hospital, I had the strangest sensation of feeling different. Was this just in my mind? Or did I actually feel it? I was changed; I knew that. My bits were gone, I was sore, as if I'd been hit by a Mack truck, and the family had functioned and managed while I was gone. What was the relevance? I don't truly know; I just know this was how I felt. It was the first week in the New Year, 2015, and here I was having limped out of hospital, now being chauffeured home.

Whilst "hubby" navigated through the suburbs, I sat back in the front seat on a comfortable foam pad and watched the world pass by me. The usual scene of cars bustling along the arterial roads and impatient drivers running red lights was not happening that day. It was school holidays and a Saturday, hence traffic was not at all congested, as that time of year, families pack up for weeks on end to escape city life and swarm the amazing coastline we have here in Queensland, either the Sunshine Coast or the infamous Gold Coast. Theme parks and water parks—every child's dream holiday is in full swing.

It was a pleasant drive, I may say. We reached the edge of suburbia and began our drive through Samford Bunya state forest. Wow, it was so nice to be amongst the tall gum trees straddling the side of the road. I wound my window down to feel the sensation of the humid heat on my face, and still managed to hear a bird or two out there singing. Nearly home! We reached the crest of the hill and began making our way down the other side, and as we neared our destination, I was able to observe through the trees snippets of rural living in the valley where we lived. As we wove down the mountain towards Samford Village, Noel asked if there was anything I wanted from the local grocery store. Keen to just get home, I answered there wasn't, but he still stopped to get the basic essentials of fresh bread and milk. That's Noel; he thinks of everything!

After he parked outside the shop, I sat quietly in the vehicle with the air-con running and reflected on the last few days. *I have gotten through it. I am nearly home.* There was relief, and yet there was still an odd sensation hovering around me. Noel returned to the car and gave me a peck on the cheek. It was like a confirmation that everything would be okay. *One day at a time, Carmel. One day at a time.*

Eight minutes past Samford Village (that is the way we measure distance out here in the country), Noel turned our wheels into our driveway. Aahh! Home sweet home! On hearing the familiar noise of the truck, Jimmy, the aged poodle, and Raffie, our ginger cat, sat beside each other behind the glass panels of the doorway patiently watching the truck edge its way up the driveway. After pulling up, Noel scooted around to my side to place the portable step in position so I could lever myself out. Jimmy, sensing that I was now home, began to whimper his traditional hello. Even though he could not see that far, if at all, he just knew that Mum was home. And Raffie, next to him, let out a meow. Oh what a lovely welcome!

Settling back in, and pet therapy

After receiving greetings from the fur kids at the front door in the foyer, I slowly made my way down the corridor and turned right into my bedroom. Standing at the door, I scanned my bedroom, pleased to be back in familiar aesthetic surroundings. In the background I could hear … nothing! Peace and quiet! No more buzzing sounds like the ones I had listened to constantly in the hospital hallways and corridors due to patients requiring attention. No more routine interruptions by hospital staff for either observation checks or meals being served. Don't get me wrong—I am so grateful for the attention to my well-being; however, in my eyes, there is nothing better than being back home where sights, sounds, and smells are familiar.

I shuffled over to my side of the bed and eased my sore and sorry body into a sitting position at the edge of the mattress. Using my hands, I raised and lifted each leg individually up onto the bed. Finally, grasping my tummy, I swung my "dead weight" around onto the bed and then slumped into the pillow. Bliss! I was home and in my own bed. No sooner had I laid my head on the pillow and started to close my eyes, then, out of the corner of my eyes, I saw that the fur kids had made their way into the room. They were sitting beside the bed looking up at me—my very overweight, PetRescue, six-year-old, female, ginger, domestic, short-hair feline, Raffie, and her pal, the gentle, quiet, timid, deaf, and quite blind, sixteen-year-old, white-and-apricot PetRescue, miniature poodle, Jimmy. They were sitting next to each other quietly observing my behaviour. I could see in their eyes the thoughts going through their minds: *Hmm, Mum doesn't look too bright!* After assessing the situation, they both leapt up onto the bed and began, in their own ways, to assess me further. Jimmy, due to his own health issues, gently manoeuvred himself up to my face. Once he located my face with his wet nose, he nudged me on the cheek and then went back to his position on my left side and snuggled into me up near my belly. Then Raffie mooched up to me, looked straight into my eyes, licked me on the cheek, and began purring. She eased back down on my right side and snuggled into me next to my tummy. In their own ways, they both acknowledged me and resumed their positions, each one choosing where each felt needed to be—beside me on opposite sides. No sooner had they cuddled into me, than the three of us dozed off for a snooze with total silence outside and a gentle breeze making its way through the open double doors.

For me, pet therapy eases overall anxiety and my emotional attachment to how I am feeling. My pets lift my mood, and they have calming effect. I remember when I took my miniature poodle Jimmy up to the aged care unit to visit my elderly parents. My father in particular responded with glee. He spent a great deal of time just lying on his bed listening to his radio, but as soon as he saw Jimmy, his eyes would light up and he would have the biggest smile. Then he would give out a big laugh and put his arms out. When I gave Jimmy to him, he would say, "Oh, Jimmy!" My dad would be just so uplifted, and happy tears would stream down his cheek.

Mum was not as responsive as my dad due to her mental health affliction and blindness; however, she would register that the dog was there and would know that it was Jimmy. When I took Jimmy up to the aged care unit, he would always coax a smile from all the residents. Whilst we were walking through the corridors on our way to my parent's rooms, the dear residents would lean out of their chairs or stop shuffling along in their wheelie walkers and ask for a pat or a cuddle. I so believe in the healing energy of being around, patting, or holding a pet. Animals just know! There is no judgement, feeling of superiority, or criticism. They offer simple, pure love and fun. When my two fur kids realized that "Mum" was not feeling 100 percent, they knew they had a job to do—just to love me.

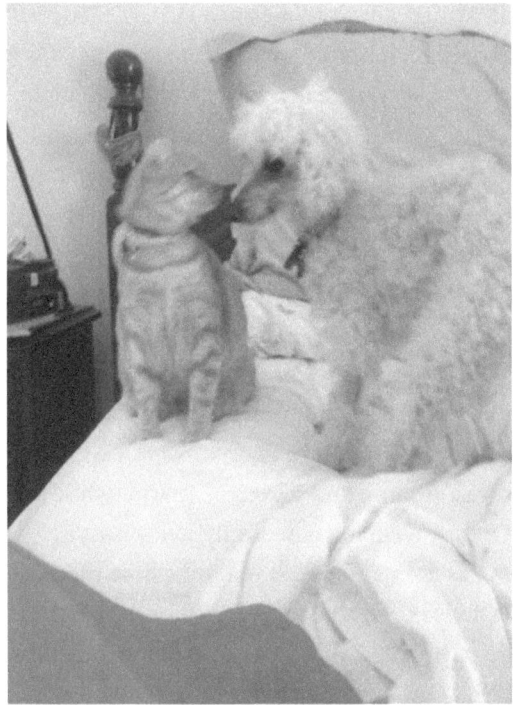

Raffie and Jimmy

One day at a time

Several days passed, and it wasn't all smooth sailing physically. The niggling pain in my side finally made itself known. I got out of bed and had incredible pain. I managed to shuffle into the ensuite to go to the loo. Something did not feel right. Sure enough—blood everywhere! *Oh, God, what is going on!*

I called out to my friend who was a houseguest at the time. As soon as I made myself respectable, we headed off to the hospital. I sat quietly back in the passenger seat thinking

I really did not want to go back to the hospital, but I really did not have any choice. I needed to resolve this nagging pain in my side, especially now that this had happened. It really had to be addressed. I had phoned the hospital and the gyno ward and told them what was happening, so they were aware that I was coming in. On arrival, as usual, we had to make our way through foyers, down lifts, and along very long corridors. As we reached the first nurses' quarters, I decided to speak to them there first, rather than having to drag my sorry body down another corridor and up another lift to where I had been originally. Making that call was obviously the right decision, as the nurse led me to an observation room and asked me to wait while she got the resident gyno. We had waited only a few minutes when the specialist came in and asked me my whole medical history for the last week. Gesturing for my houseguest to leave the room, he performed the usual intrusive check-ups. It was deemed that I would be okay to return home with another truckload of painkillers.

There was no conclusive diagnosis of what had happened. I thought it might have been the internal stitches dissolving. It also may have been something else. Gently I got down off the table, tidied myself up, and met my friend outside. We were instructed to wait for a time, as a report had to be written up for my personal specialist, and a prescription for antibiotics and painkillers had to be dispensed. Finally I was given the all-clear to leave. Off we went again toward the front entrance of the hospital. I was spent, sore, and confused by what had happened, and I had to drag myself again through corridors and in and out of lifts to reach the entrance once again of the hospital.

On the way home, I again sat quietly in the passenger seat. I felt an overwhelming feeling of sadness mixed with relief. Thoughts were passing through my mind: *What else is going to happen? How much more of this can I take?*

On reflection now, I realize this was a complete indulgence in feeling sore and sorry. There were a few quiet tears—tears of relief, cleansing, and releasing the perceived fear that there was something really wrong. It was good to have a silent cry. I just wanted to get home!

After this incident, I did feel some relief up in that area of my abdomen. The pain was not as intense as it had been from day one after the surgery. I will say, though, that the niggling pain has, even up to today, not been completely relieved. There is always a "sore sensation" there, and I am putting it down to the fact that I do need to go easy and slowly in my everyday activities and not try to do all the things I used to do before. It is so difficult, though, to remember this. However, when that pain is constant, it does bring me back to reality.

Chapter 10

Transition and Healing

Four months after the operation

$\mathcal{W}$hilst scribing my story, I thought I would check in to reconnect with the energy of my womanhood and in private. I sat down at the table and repeated the process of connecting with my body. After some quiet breaths and removing my palms from my abdomen, I gazed over the crayons, and my eyes latched onto some light, fresh colours that displayed energetic airflow. After putting crayon to paper, I was quietly taken aback by what I had drawn.

The symbolism of my uterus and ovaries was quite robust with a lot of life force energy flowing through and around. I had created the image of a strong root system anchoring my uterus, and she stood there quite upright and proud of her role as a creator and life giver. Drawing this and expressing this actually took the "edge" off the intensity of emotions that I had experienced. I was quite astounded when this happened. Perhaps it was because I had perceived in my mind that the expression in art would be less robust. I sat there looking at "her" and felt there was an energetic sense of defiance, as if she was an entity of her own. I had an amazing impression of her saying to me, "I had carried and nurtured babies. I have endured countless pap smears and countless excruciating 'flows.' I have been poked and prodded. I went through major abdominal surgery four years ago, and I am presently still standing. Physically, in the flesh, I have been removed, but my core energy will always be there for you, Carmel."

As I received this message, the tears once again welled up in my eyes. I felt the way I would if I were acknowledging and facing a death of a loved one. It was as if every fibre of my body was connected and talking together, and "she"— my "woman's bits"—already knew and had accepted the decision made. It was like the phoenix rising from the ashes! Wow, what a profound moment. Sitting motionless and digesting what had happened, I wanted to "beam" my gratitude to her through expression in words and art. I centered again and went through the ceremony of placing my palms on my abdomen, closing my eyes, and thinking about the qualities of "her" and how I would express them.

The words that came to me were *gratitude*, *respect*, *appreciation*, *astonishment*, *awe*, *beauty*, *femininity*, *passion*, *love*, *acceptance*, and *power*. On a piece of paper I wrote these words down and proceeded to express them in colour and art. Going with the flow, I immersed myself in the moment of expression. Totally absorbed by the exercise, I found myself removed from the present moment and bathing in the colour, emotion, feeling, and expression that was unfolding on paper.

What a cathartic moment! Every part of my being had experienced a shift. It was freeing, light, healing, and special. I identified that my feminine energy was still swirling through every part of my being, and that I felt connected again to all parts of myself—physical, mental, emotional, and spiritual. There was no longer self-judgement, anger, stress, sadness, grief and loss, thoughts of betrayal, disbelief and shock, or traces of being a victim.

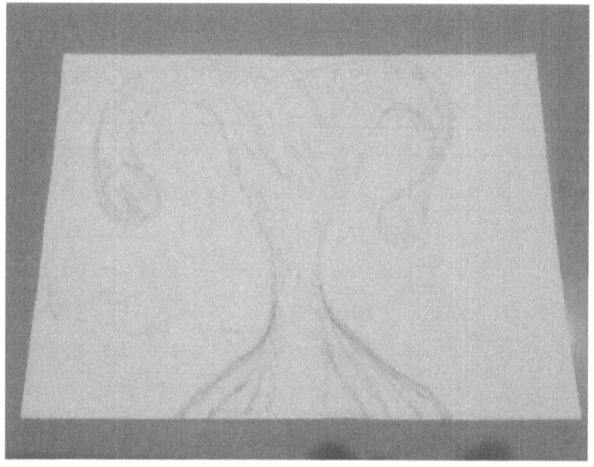

I am whole. I am beautiful. And my body, even though she bears the scars of child birth, key-hole surgery, stretch marks, and a few too many kilograms for my frame, I am amazing and still standing. The generative feminine energy of creativity, nurturing, nourishing, and passion is still there flowing and swirling through and around my abdominal area and expanding out into every cell and space of my body.

Realization struck me that I can still function without particular body parts—my uterus and ovaries, or a limb, an eye, or a breast. My experience has taught me that a healthy attitude and non-attachment to the physical—the flesh as it is in essence—is the vehicle to experience this life here on earth in the realization and reaffirmation that I am more than a physical body.

Life quality—physical wellness

Six months after my hysterectomy I observed the following:

- I physically appear to have aged more. There seems to be less elasticity in my skin, and I have a lacklustre pallor.
- My curly hair appears to have lost its bounce.
- I still become emotional and can shed a tear at the slightest sensitive thing, particularly things I see on television.
- My memory is hazy.
- My eyesight blurry.
- My stamina has waned, and I find I am not up to returning to work at full capacity. It takes me two to three days to recover from a full week of work.
- My senses are heightened but appear rational. This I had concern about, so I went to see a psychologist to discuss a particular issue that had crossed my path during and after recovery. Even though my senses were heightened, my insight and awareness were

not blurred to the extent that I read circumstances incorrectly.

• I noticed an increase in facial hair. (Ooooooo! Not happy!)

Aware that, in medical and surgical terms, my procedure had been a success, I observed that, holistically, I was still on the road of recovery. For me to return to my true self, I had to rely on my own research, taking responsibility, and continuing to talk to practitioners who could assist me to regain a holistic wellness.

I knew that, although the female reproductive organs do not produce all of the female hormones in the body, they are the major producer. And these organs had been removed. I got thinking that the loss of these organs would have ongoing consequences on my body for the rest of my life, and this would continue to influence my total well-being. This possibility did not appeal to me whatsoever. I continued to talk to other women, naturopaths, and people in the medical and pharmaceutical fields, and the question I asked frequently was, "What is the current solution to help balance and maintain a woman's body after any form of 'hyster' surgery?" I received a variety of suggestions ranging from over-the-counter herbal oral formulas, prescription hormone replacement therapy (HRT), and progesterone and estrogen creams. The alternative was to go "au naturale"; that is, do absolutely nothing, and in the process watch your well-being and sanity go down the gurgler, and witness your vitality, personality, body, and quality of life deteriorate.

The suggested alternatives all appeared to have some validation in what they did, but I questioned how I would know that I was getting complete support from any particular therapy, and what hormone was being propped up. One day I went to a girlfriend's home for lunch. Throughout our visit we were able to poke fun at ourselves as we talked about going through menopause and what an unfortunate event in a woman's life it is. We were both distressed that we, as individuals, have absolutely no control over what our bodies do and how our emotions react. "It's as if my whole self turns against me," I told her, "and I am powerless to stop it." My friend is six years younger than I, and she shared with me her concerns on beginning menopause and how it was affecting her intimacy relationship with her partner. She advised me that she had heard of a general practitioner who specialized in hormones, and hormones alone! This particular GP had done extensive research and had come up with a solution that would assist women of all ages who struggled with hormone imbalance. "Yippee!" I said. "Who is he, where is he, and when can I get into see him! Crack open the champers. I am beginning to feel an element of hope!"

This information was just what I needed to hear. As soon as I got home, I raced down the hallway to my office and jumped on my computer to Google this doctor. Gleefully, I discovered his website and felt hope rising in my chest. I excitedly scribbled down the contact number of this medical practitioner whose practice was over an hour away from where I live. One hour, two hours—who cares? I am going! My body and I are missing the hormones, and once they are balanced I won't miss the very robust cultivation of facial hair! It will be gone—soon—hopefully! I rang to make an appointment to see him the following week.

To my surprise, I was told that there was no appointment available for four months! I was gobsmacked! Being totally consumed with my challenge, I thought, *How I am going to continue on my wellness path if I have to wait another four months?* Regardless of that, I secured the appointment and thought, *In the meantime, I will continue my search for a practitioner who offers support for women with hormone woes so that I will be able to support my healing body and attempt to retain some robustness.*

So, while I awaited for my appointment with the specialist, I saw a general practitioner who worked outside the box, had an open and inquisitive mind, and included in her consultancy "alternate modalities" to complement her diagnosis. As well as Vitamin D and B12 shots, she also prescribed progesterone cream to apply at night according to the instructions. This treatment appeared to be assisting me some, and with other supportive vitamins, I felt I was beginning to feel a little better.

Finally June arrived, and I made my way north up the Bruce Highway to attend my appointment with the "hormone doctor." After the initial examination and a discussion about my written assessment of my own perception of how my body was performing, he sent me off for a comprehensive blood test that would determine my current hormone levels. A week later, I had a telephone consultation with "Dr. Hormone." He read out my own level of each hormone according to my blood test, and compared it with the ideal level. Astonishingly, my results were very poor, and for me to live and experience happy holistic health and well-being, I needed to take steps.

A brief outline of the blood tests undertaken is given below, and the results are testament that I needed hormone replacement that was personalized for my body. It was clear that a one-size-fits-all, over-the-counter treatment would not work. Keep in mind that this was my choice, and that I, within myself, knew that I felt different after my surgery. For my own well-being, I chose to investigate further and to find the best solution for my hormone health.

The blood tests determined my level of oestrogen, progesterone, testosterone, DHEA, and FSH:

- Oestrogen is ideally between 110 and 500; my level was 50.
- Progesterone is ideally between 20 and 100; my level was 5.
- Testosterone is ideally at 3; my level was 0.9.
- DHEA is ideally at 1900; my level was 1500, which was not too concerning.
- FSH should be below 30; my level was 115.

Ding! Ding! Ding! Warning bells went off in my head, mixed with elements of relief. As I had suspected, I needed extra help. I needed more hormones! I was grateful to receive the results, as now the specialist had the information he needed to prescribe a customized formula of hormones. They would be provided in the form of troches—lozenges designed to dissolve. Basically, I was in dire need of certain hormones that would assist me to begin feeling good again, and especially address the physical changes and degradation I had witnessed happening before my eyes when I looked in the mirror and bathed.

For instance, I read that oestrogen affects the brain, skin and bones, and other hormones; in fact, it is integral in the holistic wellness of a human being. My research revealed that it assists with memory loss, increases serotonin in the brain, helps maintain body temperature, and modifies production and the effect of endorphins—the feel-good hormone. As well as that, I must mention that it also assists with collagen content and quality and thickness of skin. *Yes please, I will have that!*

The next hormone I was lacking, even though I had begun, four months previously, using the therapeutic cream, was progesterone. An extremely low level was indicative of mood changes such as nervousness, anxiety, and irritability. A lack of progesterone also contributed to night sweats, weight gain, and low sex drive. (Sex drive—what's that?) There are, of course, many other symptoms of low progesterone levels in women, but these are the ones I recall experiencing.

I continued to read and learned that testosterone is something that we automatically think is a male hormone, which leads us to believe that it should not be an issue for a woman to lack this hormone. Indeed, how many of us women think that an imbalance in our testosterone level would have an impact on our hormone wellbeing? I read on the Internet that low testosterone can cause low libido, and also that the correct balance of testosterone can contribute to healthier bones. Another important fact is that balanced testosterone levels may even counteract cognitive fatigue.

I consider all of this mind-blowing information, and I ask, why is this information not readily available to each and every woman so that she can explore these options? Keep in mind, this is my story, and I am sharing the journey I went on to regain wellness. Generally, my concerns had been validated by the hormone imbalances revealed by the blood tests, and I looked forward to beginning hormone therapy to balance and regain my overall wellness—physical, mental, and spiritual.

With this information, I proceed on my personal journey of NHRT: natural hormone replacement therapy. Natural hormones are also called bio-identical or body-identical hormones. I cannot, at this stage, explain what these hormones are, as I am not a physician or bio-chemist; however, I do know that, in my heart, I prefer to use a hormone replacement that appears to be more in keeping with nature. I read on a website that the progesterone, oestrogen, and DHEA are all derived from either wild yam, clover leaf, soy beans, or other plants and herbs, and in my eyes, you cannot get more down to earth and natural than that.

At this stage of the book and my journey, I am only at the beginning of the NHRT; however, so far I am confident that this treatment will benefit me and is in line with my value choice. If, for some reason, this does not assist me, I will have to look for an alternative therapy, but for now, this is it.

Chapter 11

What Is Going On Here?

Something is not right!

*N*early five months after I began the NHRT, I noticed something was not right. The pain in my left side was not as intense, but it was always there as a constant nagging reminder. But something else had happened as well. For several days, I had begun to feel the sensation of a bulge in, or rather around, the entrance to my vagina. It felt too familiar, and my heart was beginning to sink. I felt so sullen and sad. It was uncomfortable to walk, and I had the sensation I need to "correct" myself. It felt as if the prolapse had returned. *Oh, God, no! Please, please, please let it be something else unrelated for which an invasive procedure is not required.*

I had just been getting back into the swing of my life. My income protection insurance had been denied because the assessors concluded that the hysterectomy was related to the procedure I'd had four years before. I had been unemployed, and the lack of income had been quite a strain on my partner and me. Typical of me, I was having pangs of guilt and feelings of inadequacy because I was not contributing to our household finances. I was really peeved off! It was hard not to churn it over and over in my brain, questioning myself. Had I done something to aggravate my physical health? Why had this happened? I hadn't been lifting heavy weights. I'd been doing only what my specialist said I could do—just simple housework. Surely I didn't have to go into the hospital again?

The localized sensation first appeared on the weekend, and I couldn't call my specialist for a diagnosis until Monday. As I sat writing and thinking about my situation, I just got really, really pissed off! I felt my jaw tightening and I could feel myself clenching my teeth! This just wasn't fair! I had done all the right things during the six- to eight-week recovery; I hadn't done any heavy lifting. *Why, why, why!* I was still young, energetic, and vibrant. Thoughts were going through my mind again, and I was reflecting on when this personal journey of my body, mind, and soul began and how I had the thought that there had been betrayal involved—me against myself! This wasn't supposed to happen! Not to me!

I never considered that I abused my body to the extent that I would have these problems in later years, but I had to admit that I was carrying too much weight, particularly around my abdomen, and I had not been a stickler for regular exercise. I admitted I had to take ownership of the outcome. Just processing this now, I have a sense of resolve that I do have to take some responsibility for this.

I am my body, and my body is me! Somewhere, somehow I had let it down and contributed to this potential need for further corrective surgery. As I was typing, I had a twitch in the area of my abdomen where I had been aware of the discomfort from day one. *I wonder if this has something to do with it?* I thought at the time.

I had a desire to research on the Internet to find out what needs to happen if the surgery I'd had failed, but, knowing me, if I read information that was scary, I would only upset myself more and would crawl into my pit with my doonah and have a pity party. *Avoidance! That's how I'll handle this! I'll wait until my appointment with the specialist and hear what he has to say to clarify my discomfort and concerns after the inevitable internal examination. Tomorrow, first thing, I'll call his consulting rooms and be firm that I need to see him, pronto!*

Outcome of the follow-up appointment

Wow, that was rather dramatic, wasn't it? I got an appointment right away with my specialist, and he was very understanding and comforting whilst I told him about the discomfort I was experiencing. Once again, up on the table, I had to place myself in the most unbecoming position with feet firmly planted in the "stirrups." Taking into consideration my concerns and giving me a running commentary of the surgery outcome, my specialist informed me that the surgery had been a complete success and that there was no sign of prolapse where I had been experiencing that sensation. It all appeared to be healing really well.

Okay! Well, it was really good to hear his medical perspective. I knew right there and then, though, that it would be fruitless to ask any more questions about this sensation I had been feeling, as, with no disrespect, I do not think he was able to help me. The scene was familiar yet again, but I left in a more reassured position. I paid my account, said my goodbyes, and left. Sitting in my vehicle, I thought to myself, *Well, it appears everything is where it is meant to be, and there does not appear to be any swelling. Could it be a phantom pain I am sensing? Struth! When is this all going to end?*

I decided I needed to investigate this further, just so I could experience some peace of mind. From then on, I made a mental note of everything I ate, when I evacuated, and also if I strained myself in any shape or form. This exercise of recording my activity was worthwhile. If I needed to lift something that was a little too much for me, I quickly asked someone to assist me. As well as this, I was aware that I needed to have regular bowel movements, so as to alleviate pressure in the lower parts of my body. Over time, this appears to have been the solution, and I have had not had that sensation or phantom pain again. My message here, though, is for women who have concerns about healing and recovery—do not shrug off your concern, but go and get a professional opinion. It may not be an easy solution to manage, and you may need to put yourself at ease with facts.

Six months after confirming successful surgery

Maybe I need to change my lifestyle. As I reflected on the past twelve months in relation to my challenging poor female well-being, I came to the realization that my body may be giving me a message. Maybe I wouldn't be able to go back to my career. Maybe I would have to reassess what really works for me and my body.

I did not know how I would adjust to not contributing to community as I had in my professional capacity in the field of human services. I had always been the one people came to discuss their problems. I was the one who listened. That is what I am good at; that is what makes me feel successful. Everyone has a different way of measuring success. For me it was the road I had chosen to travel down, a road that enabled me to learn, to study, to gain knowledge, and to face my own problems and issues and become a counsellor and coach. I prided myself in being approachable and empathic as I listened and, in my own way, contributed to my clients' awareness of their choices and their ability to change if they chose to do so.

Maybe that was not my path anymore. Just maybe I was to look at contributing to this life in a less demanding way and really and truly nurture myself and take it easy physically and mentally. I thought about crocheting rugs for the rest of my life through winter and continuing to do some gardening. Maybe I could actually learn to paint and draw, go to movies, have coffee with friends, and take part in all of the stress-free activities I could think of. As Noel would say, "That is not you. We will see." The man knows me so well. In fact, he cracks me up with his inner knowing and wisdom. I believe he knows me better than I know myself! He is a beautiful, caring, gentle, protective being. I am so blessed that he came into my life when, by the way, I least expected it. I was a single parent with two teenage sons and was resolved and happy to go it alone in life. The welfare and care of my boys were my priority. Anyway, I am getting off track here. Well, really, I am not, as this is all part of my life. It is part of the way disappointing health and well-being have impacted me and my family. Regardless of events and the roller-coaster ride of emotions life has thrown at me personally, my partner and my sons have been strong pillars of strength.

I decided I was not going to push myself anymore. I received no urgent message that the world would not be able to function without me. I thought I might have to consider being more domestic. Maybe I could start making healthy gluten-free cakes, and tasty snacks of vegetable stacks and hummus and the like. I could use my creativity in the kitchen rather than in a counselling room or as a workshop facilitator. I would get by. Maybe my story would resonate with other women.

Chapter 12

Activating Awareness

*I*n some capacities, we get worn down in life from the day-in-day-out routine and demands, external environment influences, pressing time frames, family responsibilities, and the like. Our life's journey is what we make it, and I am reminded that we aren't defined by our life experiences; rather, we are defined by our responses to them. I am sharing this at this stage in the book, as I want to make it known that, in the context of having this radical surgery, I strongly make this suggestion: Ladies, for your own sake, be proactive, particularly with regard to getting your hormones balanced. In addition, eat well.

During my recovery, I had a "spin out of control" reaction to a situation within my family. This caused a huge amount of awkwardness and conflict that resulted in a significant impact on the stability of some relationships. I feel that, overall, it could have been handled better by both parties; however, in saying that, I think if my hormones had been performing at healthy levels, the outcome would have been more conducive to resolution; or rather, my part in the whole "mish mash" would have been more responsible and rational rather than what it eventually deteriorated into. Yes, I put my hand up. Even people trained in counselling are human, have feelings, and are not always as composed as they could be, especially when hormones are totally compromised.

I am so grateful for the lesson my whole essence presented to me. It has reaffirmed for me that I must honour and not trivialize my feelings and emotions. It is best to acknowledge and heal the moment, but then to move forward and beyond that moment and be open to attract and receive what my "new" body can offer with more joy and ease.

Some may take longer to move through and process the emotions. It depends upon your choices, and there are no rules or limits for how long it will take to do so. On the other hand, if a loved one is aware that you appear burdened with thoughts and emotions that have not lightened up, please give yourself a fair go and respect and seek professional help to assist you out of the emotional hole you may have fallen into.

The end of our journey together

You have made it to the end of my story, and I sincerely thank you. I hope it has given you some comfort or some insight into your feelings and it has helped you to understand how each woman is an individual, and her experience is personal and unique. My aim was to contribute to your understanding of the possibilities of healing, acceptance, and what else is possible after this mind-blowing journey. There is no right or wrong way to respond. It just is! If you are going to have or have had a hysterectomy, and my experience or parts thereof rings true for you still, please be kind to yourself. Talk to your medico and seek emotional assistance through counselling or art therapy. The experience and healing will make you feel lighter and more accepting. It will help you regain the strength to move forward and silence the negative self-talk that can seep into your body, mind, and spirit.

The detrimental impact of negative energy

I thought it would be advantageous to share with you the impact of negative energy, which could be draining you. During your recovery, you need to surround yourself with folk who are capable of being supportive and who won't dump their own woes on you. Indulge yourself! You need as many hands on deck as possible to assist your recovery. Energy and emotional vampires are not welcome, thank you very much! If there is someone who is offering to help you, ask yourself this: *Is this person going to contribute to my health and recovery in a supportive and neutral manner?*

If, upon asking that question, you get a sense of "Hmmm … not really" or something similar, please do not put yourself in the position of being surrounded and trapped by that person's toxic energy. It will only contribute to a delay in your recovery.

If you are able to find family members and friends who can stay with you and support you, please allow them to look after you. A hysterectomy is a huge operation, and it impacts all facets of your being. For a period of time, your whole being is "deranged," and having support and non-judgemental help is golden.

Chapter 13

⋯⋯⋯⋯⋯❤⋯⋯⋯⋯⋯

Women from the Past—Respect and Acknowledgement

Whilst writing this dialogue about my specific challenging woman's health journey, I kept thinking of woman in the past—those who lived prior to the development of modern medicine. One of these women is my dear mother who is now eighty-seven years old. Due to challenging needs, she is now living in amazingly caring aged care facility. Even though Mum has signs of dementia, I am blessed that she still recognizes me when I visit, and when we talk over the phone at times, we can still have conversations relating to the present as well as the past. Every couple of days as I was writing this book, I would phone Mum and discuss my progress, and she, in her feminine wisdom, would give me advice on how to care for myself. One day she said, "It is a major operation, Carmel, and you need to really look after yourself. Are you wearing support panties? Remember to place your hand on your tummy so as not to strain yourself."

Numerous times mum experienced traumatic female health reproductive issues similar to me. Whilst chatting to my mum just the other day, she told me that she was having a hot Milo. As she sipped, I told her that I wanted to acknowledge the incredible strength, courage, and resilience she had demonstrated back in those days. I let her know it was amazing how she had come through it all emotionally reasonably well (for a time … but more in a moment). Mum responded in a matter of fact way. "Way back then, Carmel, our emotions and all of that were just swept under the carpet."

Wow, how profound! Emotions were swept under the carpet back then! Has it really changed or improved much since then? Keeping this in perspective, I am referring to the emotional upset of a hysterectomy and miscarriage here, as I can speak only on behalf of what I have gone through personally and nothing else. Getting back to Mum's response regarding her emotional resilience, it was not so long ago, as her memory diminished, that she experienced quite a few meltdowns regarding the loss of her miscarried babies. Suddenly, her grief and loss all came pouring out. Brutally, emotional pain appeared to have been embedded in her memory more than fifty years later.

If a woman who is prone to feel such depth of emotion does not receive professional help, does she ever get over these experiences or learn to live with them? Without any kind of healing, when the pain of that old wound seeps through the sands of time, that woman has to do her own sweeping of the emotion under the carpet in silence.

I have spoken to many women about this topic, and I have received a variety of responses. Some women do connect totally to what I am saying, and empathy and recognition is written all over their faces. Other women acknowledge that they, too, have had a hysterectomy, and from their voice tone and body language, I sense that they adopted a "suck-it-up" attitude and appeared to have an expectation that everyone else in the same situation should suck it up as well. One particular woman I spoke to was the manager of a local obstetrician/gynaecologist's practice. Her manner towards me was quite remarkable to say the least. I had called on a number of "gynos" that day to share my thoughts about the perceived lack of emotional support for women enduring a hysterectomy. Each time, I gave my "elevator pitch" calmly and slowly. I offered my observation to this woman and told her how I was offering specific emotional support to hysterectomy patients. But before I could finish my sentence, she basically cut me off. Yep, she wanted me out of the reception area—pronto!

Why would someone in that position respond like that? What if there was a patient sitting in the reception area eavesdropping on our conversation? How would anyone know how that woman was feeling? Whatever the reason was for her behaviour, it was to me a reflection of my mum's comment that all the emotion had been "swept under the carpet." How grim!

So I, with reverence and respect, acknowledge all women in every country, creed, and race from the past as well as women from the present and the future who have endured and who will endure the trauma of the physical removal and disconnection of their reproductive organs in a partial or full hysterectomy. I also revere and respect those who miscarry and those who have no choice fall pregnant whether they choose to or not. My heart goes out to you all with complete empathy and as much understanding I have to share from my own journey.

In my head I hear the lyrics written by Helen Reddy and Ray Burton and performed by Reddy: "I am Woman." This song reflects how strong we women really are; even through all kinds of adversity we are still standing. In the context of my subject in this book, we are still reproducing; we are still mothers, sisters, aunts, maidens, cousins, and active career women, sports women and more, contributing to all of life, each in our own personal way. Let's support each other as much as we can.

Chapter 14

―――●○♥○●―――

What Now?

*W*ell, we have come to the end of my personal story. I have recounted my experience in its complete, personal, raw form, and you, the reader, have been drawn into my private and personal abode—my very body, mind, and spirit. Together we have both survived the incredible bumpy, emotional, and sometimes tragic scenes, and we are still standing. For me the writing has been a cathartic experience, and my reflections have given me an overwhelming appreciation for the female body—her form and the sacred awesomeness of what she is and what she can create. *Struth, girls, we are good!*

From a layperson's perspective, I am indeed humbled by the greatness of our Creator who, in his, her, or its universal wisdom, power, and magnificence created all humans, and in particular the complex female reproductive organs. From this experience, I will continue to be an advocate for the physical and emotional healing and well-being of all women who are faced with any form of hysterectomy, and I will continue to spread the word that the whole person experiences and is impacted by reactive emotions when it involves any part of her body. We relate to our bodies and minds as one. For me it is duality, and for success there must be a bridging of the separateness and even more acknowledgement that the emotions and mental health of a woman who is having a hysterectomy impacts her healing.

Since I began writing and sharing my experience, I have taken steps to promote awareness about the need and importance of emotional support for women who are recovering from any type of hysterectomy or procedure involving her reproductive system.

I have organized promotional stalls at Women's Health and Wellbeing Expo at Morayfield as well at the local district Samford Health and Wellness Expo. At both events, women have come up to me and shared their stories. I learned that, evidently, some of them are still reeling emotionally as well as physically from the trauma. With such reinforcement of my own conviction, I felt I needed to raise the awareness. I then made a list of the majority of gynaecologists in the metropolitan area of SE Queensland, Australia, and I sent out e-mails to raise the emotional awareness. I even "hit the road" and knocked on the doors of many specialists. I spoke with their practice managers of my personal experience and my emotional rollercoaster.

I have been successful in being invited to speak to a group of gynaecologists/obstetricians at a local hospital and medical training facility. At first I had some trepidation; however, when I began sharing my story, I will admit my passion and conviction began to pump through my veins. I am hopeful that speaking with them will raise their awareness that emotional support must be part of the healing of a woman's body, both pre- and post-op.

So there we go, folks. I have laid my whole experience out on the table for the world to read and see. I truly hope sharing my experience reassures you that you are not going mad. You are not silly. What you are feeling is real, and that there is support out there somewhere. Ask questions—many questions. Take your recovery slowly. Be kind to yourself. And when there are kind people offering to help, please receive it!

Peace be with you,

Carmel

Art Therapy Activities

Gather together the following resources to use in the healing activities in this chapter:

- Crayons, paints, coloured pencils, markers … whatever you like to work with
- Plain sheets of paper, any size you like
- Candles
- A pretty scarf or cloth
- Any representative objects you wish to use in your symbolic gesture ceremony; for example, a flower to represent a garden or a teddy bear to represent childhood
- A box of tissues
- A table and a comfortable chair

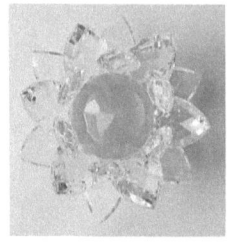

Healing Activity One: *Acknowledging and connecting with your reproductive organs*

- Sit quietly with your back comfortably upright, feet on the floor, and your eyes gently closed.
- Lay the palms of your hands gently on your abdomen approximately where your reproductive organs are.
- Breathe in and out slowly to become centred and relaxed.
- To assist yourself to connect with that area through your breathing, think of a colour that you relate to and visually breathe in that colour. It may be any colour that comes to you and feels like the colour you need.
- You can also draw on the colour orange, which is the sacral colour chakra of the chakra system, the life-force energy system. It is said that this area of the body is connected to feelings of sensitivity, joy, happiness, and the inner child; hence, if that is the case, no wonder after a partial or full hysterectomy, emotions are in overload. Connecting to energy healing can only assist.
- Visualize the coloured breath making its way down to the reproductive area and cycling through, in, and around the organs.
- With your breathing, send words of particular meaning to you and your body. During your centred breathing, words of quality may come to you. They could be messages of essence: Thank you. I love you. I am grateful. Blessings.

- During this activity, emotions may rise. Continue gentle breathing; give allowance to your reaction, being present with acknowledgement and honour.
- If there are tears, when they subside and your breathing is regular, gently open your eyes and bring yourself to the room, taking in the sounds and surroundings.

Healing Activity Two:
A continuation of healing activity one

Activity One alone will begin to shift energy through your body and provide you with a growing awareness of your emotional rawness. To assist with the energetic healing of your whole being—body, mind, and spirit—the next step is to bring in positive, nurturing thoughts and words and express them through colour, shapes, symbolism, free drawing, or whatever way resonates to you.

Here are the qualities I drew on that related to my own reproductive system. Each point has a deep meaning for me:

- Gratitude
- Unconditional love
- Awe
- Miraculous creative power
- Safe nurturing incubator
- I am part of you, and you are a part of me
- Generative energetic force
- Beauty of the feminine

I shared my art expression of these qualities in Chapter Ten. As I created, the artwork took on a life of its own. I gazed over my box of oil-based crayons, and the first colour that jumped out at me was purple. Shades of pink and red followed. The large nucleus expressed the miraculous creative power and potency of incubation that my body was capable of achieving. The generative energy life force had the endurance every month of developing and producing ova on the chance that one of them might become fertilized. Whilst I was absorbed in drawing my expression of qualities, I was awakened to awareness of how awesome a woman's body is.

I sat for some time just feeling connected to the art piece, breathing in the colour qualities I had just expressed. There was a feeling of lightness about me and a renewed gratitude for the beauty and potency of my own body—and indeed the bodies of all women. I then felt the urge to stand and gesture and move my body like the flow of energy in my drawing. As I did this, I felt connected even more and could feel the energy lightly pump through my body and limbs. It was a truly lovely personal healing experience.

- Find a quiet, private space where you feel comfortable—either outside or in your home.
- Have in front of you your art paper and crayons, pencils, markers, or paints.
- Sit quietly centred with the intention of soothing, nurturing, and acknowledging your womanhood.
- Allow your mind's eye to sense within and to bring to your attention the qualities that relate to you and to your relationship with your reproductive organs.

- Jot down each word that springs to your mind and see if you can relate that word to a colour or symbol.
- Give yourself the time and space to express each quality in free-spirited art expression.
- Become immersed in the flow of expression, and make a mental note of the feeling or emotion you connected with the exercise.
- Grab a notepad and record this experience, which is reflected in your art.
- If you wish, step back from the piece and gesture your appreciation, either in words, hand gestures, dance, or quiet prayer.
- When you are ready, acknowledge this sacred time and space and give yourself permission to move forward.

Healing Activity Three:
Healing, honour, and closure ceremony

Prepare an altar of gratitude and release:

- Locate a quiet, private space in your home.
- Set up a small table. A coffee table, sideboard, or any flat, raised space can serve as an altar.
- Cover the surface with a ceremonial cloth. It can be a scarf, a throw rug, or even an item of clothing that resonates with you.
- Arrange your drawings of therapeutic healing on top of the cloth, or around the altar if they are large.

- Select from your belongings the items that you would like to place on your altar. They should relate intimately with you and your theme.
- Place candles where you are drawn to on the cloth, making sure they are well away from anything that is flammable.

Prepare the words to be said:

- You may want to use the words I used in my personal ceremony, which I have included here, or you may want to write your own words, which may have more significance to you.
- Set the mood with dim lighting and soft, relaxing music in the background. Give thanks and release your physical attachment to your reproductive system. Here are my own words: "To my woman's bits—for all these years, I have been a part of you, and you have been a part of me, there have been trying times with unbearable discomfort and pain, and yet I am grateful …"
- After reciting your personal, heartfelt words, sit quietly with this energy for a while, allowing the specialness of the moment wash over you. When you are ready to leave this moment, having said all you wanted to say, take a deep breath, blow out the candles, stretch gently, and, in a final gesture, bow or clasp your hands together in front of your heart signalling the end of the ceremony.
- If it is convenient, you may want to leave your altar on display for a while, for as long as you wish. There

is no right or wrong way to do this. You will know if and when you wish to disassemble the altar of honour of your women's bits.

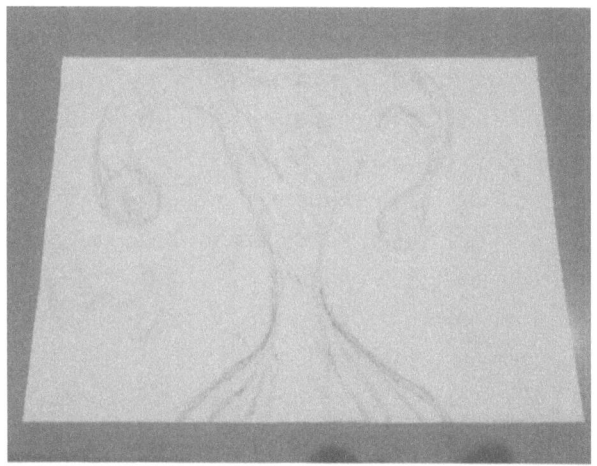

Message and Expression

"I have carried and nurtured babies. I have endured countless pap smears and countless excruciating 'flows.' I have been poked and prodded. I went through major abdominal surgery four years ago, and I am presently still standing. Physically, in the flesh, I have been removed, but energetically I will still be there for you, Carmel."

The words that came to me were *gratitude*, *respect*, *appreciation*, *astonishment*, *awe*, *beauty*, *feminine*, *passion*, *love*, *acceptance*, and *power*.

Healing Activity Four: *Personal spiritual belief preparation on the day of surgery*

- On being admitted to hospital, ask for or find some quiet time on your own so you can rest in prayer or meditation. A private room is ideal if that is possible, but you can find the mental space even just lying in your hospital bed.
- Acknowledge the connection of your spirit (the soul, the higher self, the infinite being) to your God (the creator, the divine)
- Pray or meditate for protection and courage as you face the medical procedure.
- Pray for and bless the surgeon, anaesthetist, and theatre staff so that they will be professional, open, hygienic, and safety conscious at all times.
- On being taken into the theatre, connect with your creator in prayer and ask for protection and honour for the sacred space of your body.
- Bless the theatre room with love. Visualize the theatre bathed in healing white energy and love.
- Visualize all the equipment and implements bathed in your creator's divine love and protection.
- During prep, before going under anaesthesia, recite the Lord's Prayer or any prayer or verse of your choosing, asking for respectful conversation and reference to your sacred body during the operation by all theatre staff.
- When you are ready, take a cleansing breath and relax.

List of Aussie Slang

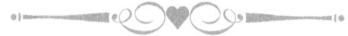

B!**dy	a curse word
brekkie	breakfast
champers	champagne
chook	chicken
doonah	bed quilt, comforter
ensuite	a bathroom that is directly connected to a bedroom
gobsmacked	astounded
gyno	gynaecologist
hyster	hysterectomy
loo	bathroom, toilet
medico	medical professional

Milo	brand name for a malted chocolate drink
mish mash	mixed bag, muddled up
mobie	mobile phone
Norman Gunsten	An Australian comedy character, who from shaving had nicks and cuts all over his face and who had bits of tissue on each cut to stop the bleeding.
peeved off	angered
Perspex®	acrylic
rig	platform, type of crane
skerrick	the smallest bit
struth	expression of surprise
wardsman	orderly (in a hospital)

www.ingramcontent.com/pod-product-compliance
Lightning Source LLC
Chambersburg PA
CBHW020536290526
45786CB00002B/908